Medicine Demystified

(Volume 1)

The Regeneration Promise: The Facts behind Stem Cell Therapies

Authored By

Professor Peter Hollands

Freelance Consultant Clinical Scientist
Huntingdon, Cambs PE261LB
UK

Medicine Demystified

(Volume 1)

The Regeneration Promise: The Facts behind Stem Cell Therapies

Author: Peter Hollands

ISBN (Online): 978-981-14-8213-7

ISBN (Print): 978-981-14-8211-3

ISBN (Paperback): 978-981-14-8212-0

need for a court order if at any point you breach any terms of this License Agreement. In no event will any delay or failure by Bentham Science Publishers in enforcing your compliance with this License Agreement constitute a waiver of any of its rights.

3. You acknowledge that you have read this License Agreement, and agree to be bound by its terms and conditions. To the extent that any other terms and conditions presented on any website of Bentham Science Publishers conflict with, or are inconsistent with, the terms and conditions set out in this License Agreement, you acknowledge that the terms and conditions set out in this License Agreement shall prevail.

Bentham Science Publishers Pte. Ltd.
80 Robinson Road #02-00
Singapore 068898
Singapore
Email: subscriptions@benthamscience.net

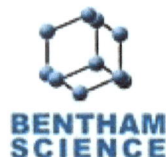

CONTENTS

PREFACE

The aim of this book is to bring a clear understanding and appreciation of stem cell technology and the related subject of regenerative medicine to everyone and especially to those people considering paying for stem cell therapy or stem cell related services. It avoids complex scientific terminology (or it is clearly and simply defined where needed) and develops ideas in a coherent and understandable fashion for the general reader.

The subject of stem cell technology and the related possible regenerative medicine procedures is an area of science and medicine where there is much confusion, often supported by unproven claims. There are currently many clinics offering stem cell 'treatments' which are driven by profit with no concern for the safety or well-being of the patient. There are untested and unproven stem cell based 'treatments' being offered to vulnerable patients around the globe and these are often sold at a very high price. If these 'treatments' were offered free of charge, it would still be scandalous behaviour by those offering such treatments because the 'treatments' are untested and unproven and could even pose a health risk to vulnerable, often terminally or acutely ill recipient patients.

The general public, who are the people most likely to consider, or to be offered stem cell-based therapies, in most instances often have little or no understanding of stem cell technology and put their trust in 'clinic' salesmen.

This is not the fault of the patients, it is the fault of those people who wish to draw such patients into a web of deceit.

The salesmen who represent the clinics often have no knowledge or formal training in stem cell technology at all and are all driven by profit. The result of this is that vulnerable patients, who may be suffering from life threatening or life changing diseases, are drawn into costly stem cell procedures which are at best unproven and could sometimes even be damaging rather than beneficial to their health. This must stop. This book will give everyone the knowledge to assess and reject such 'treatments' if they are inappropriate. Patients must be prepared to walk away if they have any doubts about the safety and efficacy of any proposed treatment and if a treatment does commence, it must always be under informed consent.

It is not just the general public and potential patients who need stem cell information. Many practising physicians have had little or no stem cell training in medical school, most journalists have no knowledge at all in the subject and politicians make life changing decisions on the use and availability of stem cell technology often based on a very poor level of understanding. The book will also be a useful resource to students both in school and University who want to begin their understanding of stem cell technology and become the stem cell pioneers of the future. Thorough training of our future physicians, scientists and businessmen in stem cell concepts will help resolve the problems we currently have in the clinical application of stem cell technology. The problem which we see today in stem cell technology, and the related regenerative medicine, is considerably magnified by the patient's vulnerability, confusion, fear and blind trust in an atmosphere where the unwary can lose not only lots of money but also potentially their health.

The Regeneration Promise offers truly new and thorough insight into stem cell technology and it is written in a style that anyone can easily understand. There is no complex terminology (except where absolutely needed and if the terminology is used then it is carefully explained) and the stem cell concepts are described in a simple and accessible style that can be enjoyed and understood by all readers. The book is aimed at the general public, potential patients, physicians, students, journalists and anyone with a general interest in stem cell technology. No specialist knowledge is needed, and most importantly the information the book contains is evidence based and has no bias or hidden agenda. The Regeneration Promise is therefore a reliable and trusted point of reference for anyone either interested in stem cells or considering treatment using stem cells.

CONSENT FOR PUBLICATION

Not applicable.

CONFLICT OF INTEREST

The authors declare no conflict of interest, financial or otherwise.

ACKNOWLEDGEMENTS

Declared none.

Peter Hollands
Freelance Consultant Clinical Scientist
Cambridge, UK
E-mail: peterh63@hotmail.com

DEDICATION

This book is dedicated to my partner Louise Barrett for her love, dedication and support. I must also thank my cardiac surgeon Mr. Ian Wilson and everyone at Liverpool Heart and Chest Hospital without whom none of this would be possible!

CHAPTER 1

A Bit of History

(An overview of the historical development of stem cell technology from 1956 to the present day)

A small body of determined spirits fired by an unquenchable faith in their mission can alter the course of history.
Mahatma Gandhi

Summary: This introductory chapter provides a general overview of the history of the development of the understanding of stem cell technology and the importance of stem cells to us all in everyday life. It provides important information on the basic science behind stem cell technology and it is an important foundation for readers to enjoy and understand the rest of the book.

INTERESTING TIMES

The year 1956 was interesting in many ways. Post-war recovery was progressing very well and new technology was being developed and brought into the home and the work place to make everyday lives easier and more productive. In the UK, luxuries such as the washing machine and vacuum cleaner were revolutionising the domestic role of women and optimism was high with the ending of rationing and a general post-war euphoria. In the Middle East, however, the 'Suez Crisis' brought great tension with Britain and France being drawn into military conflict in the area and Castro started a revolution in Cuba. Meanwhile, the first transatlantic telephone cable became operational while a young man called Elvis Presley was singing about his 'Blue Suede Shoes'. It was, therefore, a year of some stress (not least dirty blue suede shoes), but at the same time, this was balanced by a 'feel good' factor perhaps enhanced by the newly discovered psychedelic drugs such as LSD and derivatives which would go on to dominate 'flower power' in the 1960's. 1956 was also very important in the development of the understanding and clinical use of stem cells. Before we go any further with these ideas, it is necessary to properly understand what stem cells are and why they are important to us.

STEM CELLS ARE EVERYWHERE!

Stem cells are present in every human being, mammal and some reptiles and no doubt will eventually be found in all species in some shape or form. Stem cell science is in its' infancy and much more research is needed to come even close to an understanding of the importance and potential of stem cells. We can, however, be very certain that stem cells are essential for our normal development, normal health and possibly our ageing and eventual death. Stem cells may have been around since the first development of life on planet Earth (probably around 4.1 billion years ago) and no doubt exist in various types of life forms on other planets that are yet to be discovered (stem cells but not as we know it!).

Even in the early 21st century, we still have a lot to learn about stem cell biology and how we can manipulate stem cells to our benefit for our general health, treatment of disease and treatment of accidents such as spinal damage or burns. The unique properties of stem cells enable them to repair and regenerate tissue in our bodies for the whole of our lifespan which first develop in the early embryo at the very beginning of life. When stem cells go wrong then they can become the basis of very serious diseases such as leukaemia and cancer and understanding the nature of these 'tumour forming' stem cells will lead to a better understanding of how tumours arise and how they may be prevented or treated.

Bone Marrow Stem Cells

The most studied human stem cells to date are found in the bone marrow. Bone marrow is found inside the large bones of our skeleton, such as the thigh bone and the pelvis (hip bone). Bone marrow stem cells were the first stem cells to be discovered following many years of research on mouse bone marrow. These bone marrow stem cells in humans are capable of producing 200 billion red cells (these carry oxygen into the body and carbon dioxide out of the body), 10 billion white cells (these fight infection) and 400 billion platelets (these help to produce clots when needed) *per day*. The bone marrow stem cells are therefore known as 'blood forming' stem cells and without them blood, and therefore human life, would not exist in its present form. This astonishing feat by bone marrow stem cells means that just over 2000 red cells, just over 1000 white cells and just over 4000 platelets are produced *every second* in every one of us! This is biology at its' most efficient and elegant state and we still have lots to learn about the process of forming blood, which is a remarkable process starting in the very early human embryo and carrying on until death.

The figures given above on blood cell production by bone marrow stem cells illustrate the importance of stem cells in our normal healthy lives and the enormous potential for problems when stem cells go wrong. The stem cells in the bone marrow are truly amazing but no less so than, for example, stem cells in skin which repair and rejuvenate our skin on a daily basis and stem cells in the whole of the gastrointestinal tract (mouth to anus) which repair and maintain the cells of this vital organ. Human life would be impossible without stem cells and when stem cells either stop working or become diseased then the consequences can be severe and sometimes even deadly.

Back Again to 1956

Getting back to 1956, the significant thing which happened this year in stem cell technology was the first human bone marrow stem cell transplant in the world. Dr E. Donnal 'Don' Thomas in the USA and his team were the pioneers and the patient was an identical twin who received bone marrow from her identical sibling. Identical twins have identical genetics, which means that tissue or cells can be transplanted from one twin to the other twin without any worry of rejection of the donated tissue or cells. The recipient patient twin would have been treated with chemotherapy (drugs which destroy cancer) and radiotherapy (X rays which destroy cancer) prior to the transplant. The donor twin would have undergone a bone marrow harvest under general anaesthetic to obtain the bone marrow stem cells for transplantation. Unlike a tissue transplant, such as a kidney transplant or heart transplant, bone marrow stem cells are transplanted to the recipient patient using the intravenous route (directly into a vein). This highlights an amazing feature of bone marrow stem cells: They can be injected into a vein and they find their way to the bone marrow where they 'set-up home' and begin making blood cells. This 'homing' of stem cells is a very useful property and is often utilised in stem cell transplants to other tissue where tissue specific stem cells can 'home' to the area of damage or disease and begin their repair process.

In 1990, Don Thomas and his colleague Joseph E. Murray were awarded the Nobel prize for their pioneering work in bone marrow stem cell transplantation. Better late than never!

Tissue Typing or 'Tissue Matching'

These early bone marrow transplants were soon followed by a clear understanding in 1968 of the importance of 'matching' donor and recipient or this matching is also called tissue typing or Human Leucocyte Antigen (HLA) typing. Donors and recipients of bone marrow can be 'matched' to avoid or minimise 'rejection' or what is technically known as graft *versus* host disease (GvHD). This work was carried out by Dr. Jean Dausset and his colleagues Dr George Snell and Dr Baruj Benacerraf. These three scientists shared the Nobel prize for their work on tissue typing in transplantation in 1980. Once again better late than never!

The understanding of tissue typing meant that donor and recipient could be matched as far as possible, and therefore, the chances of rejection are considerably reduced. This made the whole process of bone marrow transplantation safer. This recognition of both Dr Don Thomas and Dr Jean Dausset and their colleagues by the Nobel committee illustrates the critical importance of their ground-breaking work, which is still the basis of many stem cell transplants today.

Nevertheless, rejection (or GvHD) can be fatal for some transplant patients so understanding and applying this knowledge was a very important step in the development of safe bone marrow stem cell transplantation to unrelated patients. This advance meant that bone marrow stem cells could be transplanted between unrelated people with relative safety assuming that a 99-100% match between donor and recipient can be found. This has resulted in over 1 million bone marrow stem cell transplants globally to date and these transplants often used bone marrow stem cells obtained from large international public stem cell banks such as Anthony Nolan in the UK or the New York Stem Cell Foundation.

This success in using bone marrow as a source of stem cells for transplantation marked the beginning of many years of stem cell research, extending to the present day, which in turn has made us aware of many different types of stem cells which exist in the body and their importance and potential. There will no doubt be many further discoveries in stem cell technology in the years to come, but the progress and innovation since 1956 and up to today have been beyond all expectations and let us hope that this momentum continues.

From Embryos to Stem Cells

The next important player in the stem cell story is Professor Sir Robert Edwards (known as Bob to his friends and colleagues) who worked at Cambridge University in the Physiological Laboratory (The Marshall Laboratory) and was a Fellow of Churchill College, Cambridge. Bob is much better known for his work in IVF (test-tube babies) as the pioneer of this technology, along with his physician colleague Mr Patrick Steptoe. Bob received the Nobel prize for his work on IVF in 2010. Unfortunately, Patrick Steptoe had died by the time the Nobel prize was awarded and therefore could not receive the award posthumously. Both Patrick and Bob can be seen in Fig. (**1**) which was at the first meeting of the European Society of Human Reproduction and Embryology (ESHRE) in Bonn in 1985. They were both dear friends, colleagues and mentors of mine and they are sadly missed by myself and hundreds of thousands of colleagues and patients around the World.

Getting back to stem cells, in the 1960's to the Noughties Bob Edwards wrote some very important papers about stem cell technology with an amazing insight and understanding of what was happening at the time and what may happen in the future. His focus was on stem cell development in the early embryo and his ideas were the inspiration for me when I carried out research for my PhD at Cambridge University with Bob as my supervisor. Bob died in 2013 but his legacy in IVF and stem cell technology lives on today in every baby born by assisted reproduction and in concepts and developments in regenerative medicine.

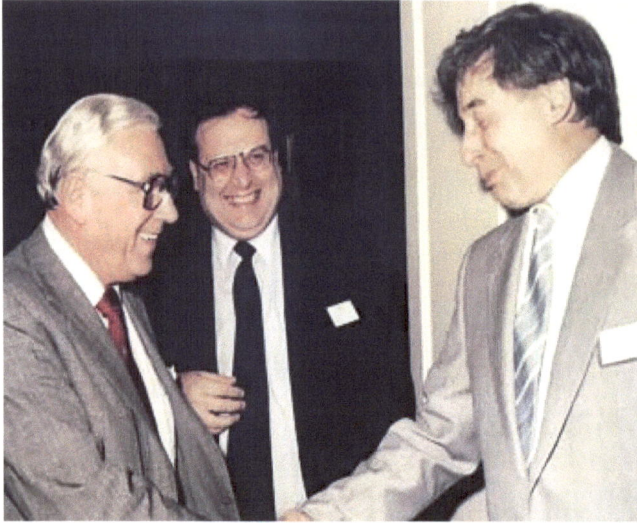

Fig. (1). Bob Edwards (on the right) and Patrick Steptoe (on the left) at the first meeting of the European Society of Human Reproduction and Embryology (ESHRE) in Bonn. I presented the stem cell work from my PhD at this meeting.

From Mouse to Man?

It was the early 1980's when a very handsome and intelligent young student, supervised by Bob Edwards, started research work to identify stem cells in the early mouse embryo (just after the mouse embryo has implanted into the uterus) and to attempt to use these cells to treat blood disease in other mice. Three years of research showed that there were indeed stem cells in the early mouse embryo and that these cells could be easily extracted and used to treat other mice suffering from blood disorders with great success. I created a very simple diagram of the basis of my work and made it into a 35mm slide, (Fig. **2**). This slide travelled the World with Bob Edwards when he talked about my research at international conferences. It is perhaps one of the significant moments in regenerative medicine leading to some of the work and concepts we see today.

The research also confirmed the extraordinary properties of stem cells in the developing embryo which seemed to be capable of crossing transplant barriers such as tissue type and producing donor cells at an amazing rate. Cynics might say that this is good news if you happen to be a mouse and they are in part correct. Taking such ideas and technology from mouse to man is a massive and expensive technological and logistical task which I will cover later. Nevertheless, the results were still interesting to the overall understanding of the rapidly developing field of stem cell technology and earned me a PhD from Cambridge University! I thank the mice without whom this knowledge would have been impossible to obtain, they are all heroes.

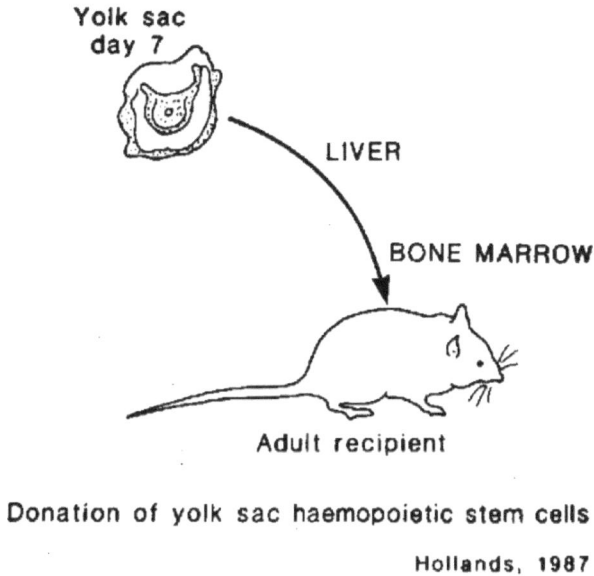

Fig. (2). A basic 35mm slide of my work, drawn by me, which Bob Edwards used in many international conferences.

In terms of Bob Edwards and IVF it is also interesting to note that sperm production is driven by stem cells in the adult testis. This is unlike the limited total number of eggs in a human female where no egg stem cells are present to replenish egg numbers. The presence of sperm stem cells (known technically as spermatogonia) in the testis results in the ability of a male to produce sperm, and potentially father children, for the whole of his adult lifetime. Sperm stem cells are today a subject of intense research as people try to understand and treat male infertility which is on the rise in the World.

More Mouse Embryos!

In 1981, another Cambridge academic, Professor Sir Martin Evans and his colleagues, described the first preparations of stem cells from mouse embryos *before* implantation in the uterus (unlike my own work which focussed on embryos after implantation in the uterus) and this resulted in yet another Nobel prize in 2007! This was considered to be a very important development because mouse embryonic stem cells were a new classification of stem cells which can produce most of the tissues in the body (known scientifically as pluripotent stem cells) and not just blood cells as described for bone marrow. Momentum was now really building up in the identification of different types of stem cells and because of the mouse stem cell discoveries many people started to talk about potentially treating a whole range of disease and physical damage (known scientifically as pathology and trauma respectively) with stem cells. This is the foundation of what we know today as Regenerative Medicine and is the subject of much hope and excellent research but at the same time, in some instances, much hype, misinformation and even scientific fraud!

Stem Cells in The Blood

The excellent initial work on bone marrow stem cell transplantation was further refined in 1981 when technology was developed to collect stem cells from the peripheral blood (veins) rather than bone marrow. This was a major step forward because a bone marrow harvest for transplant is a relatively painful procedure carried out under a general anaesthetic. The bone marrow is collected from the hip bone of the donor and there is often pain and bruising as a result plus the risk of receiving a general anaesthetic and bleeding and infection following the procedure. Dr J.M. Goldman and his colleagues discovered that it is possible to make stem cells come out of the bone marrow into the peripheral circulation (blood in the veins) by using medication. These bone marrow stem cells in the peripheral blood can then be collected using a process called 'apheresis' which is a very clever centrifuge. The donor is attached to the apheresis machine, by a highly trained nurse or apheresis scientist, and the stem cells are extracted from the donor blood. The rest of the blood cells and plasma go back to the donor after going through the apheresis machine. The stem cells which have been collected are then processed and frozen in liquid nitrogen so that they are ready for the recipient. These peripheral blood stem cells are most usually returned to the original patient after treatment has removed all disease. Such a process is often used in some diseases to collect stem cells from a patient suffering from a blood disease, treat the patient for the disease, and then return the original stem cells back to the original patient. This is known as an autologous transplant and it has become increasingly important in the routine treatment of blood disorders. This use of peripheral blood autologous stem cell transplantation was the original approach used by Dr. Goldman and his team.

This process of collection of peripheral blood stem cells by apheresis made bone marrow stem cell donation easier and it has now become the stem cell collection method of choice for a wide range of leukaemia and related blood disorders. As a result of this improved method of collecting bone marrow stem cells from the circulation there are very few 'traditional' bone marrow collections carried out today with the first line choice for most transplant physicians being peripheral blood stem cells.

Cord Blood Stem Cells

The next important development in blood forming stem cell technology came from an unexpected source when in 1988 the first ever cord blood stem cell transplant was announced. This achievement was the culmination of about ten years previous research into cord blood which remains in the umbilical cord and placenta when a baby is born. It was discovered that this cord blood contains 'blood forming' stem cells and this led to the idea that these cord blood stem cells could possibly be used in a transplant in a similar way to bone marrow stem cells.

The first ever cord blood transplant, carried out in Paris by Dr. Eliane Gluckman and her colleagues, was used to treat a little boy aged 5 suffering from a type of inherited genetic anaemia. The donor in this case was the newborn sister of the little boy and the patient, Matthew Farrow, is alive and well today as a result of receiving his new born sisters' cord blood in a transplant. The use of cord blood as a source of stem cells has become a popular treatment method for leukaemia and blood disorders and there have been over 40,000 transplants to date for over 80 different blood diseases (this is pretty much every blood disease known!).

Cord blood can be collected and stored by private cord blood banks who store the cord blood for a fee and it is then kept for the use of the family only. It can also be collected and stored by public cord blood banks where cord blood is donated and made available for transplant to anyone in need. These concepts relating to private and public cord blood collection and storage will be discussed in detail later in Chapter 4.

Cord Blood Transfusion

Cord blood has also been proposed and proven, by my dear friend and colleague Professor Niranjan Bhattacharya in Calcutta India, as a possible alternative or supplement to donated adult blood for transfusion. The use of cord blood as a transfusion product has been shown to be safe and effective for patients who need a blood transfusion when suffering from both disease and trauma. This concept could save lives globally, maintain a totally reliable source of valuable blood for transfusion and save hospitals and health care providers considerable amounts of money by reducing recovery times of transfusion recipients. The challenge here is to get people to accept this life saving technology and this will be discussed later in the book.

All of the clinical transplants and the transfusions mentioned above have used 'blood forming' stem cells found in the bone marrow and umbilical cord blood. These stem cells can make all of the cells in the blood which as described earlier are red cells, white cells and platelets. I have mentioned the discovery of mouse embryonic stem cells but of course these had no role in the treatment of humans but did spur researchers on to seek out the possibility of human embryonic stem cells in human embryos.

Human Embryonic Stem Cells

During my time as one of the first clinical embryologists in the world, working in the early 1980's at the first ever IVF clinic at Bourn Hall in the Cambridgeshire countryside, I would look down the microscope and see human embryos develop. Their beauty and symmetry were amazing. It was an awe inspiring and privileged sight to be one of the first human beings to see the start of human life. When we looked at these embryos Bob Edwards and I knew that these human embryos must contain stem cells and that one day, in theory, these stem cells could possibly be used to treat disease and to repair tissue. A typical human blastocyst, which is probably one of the first images of this kind taken by myself at Bourn Hall Clinic, is shown in Fig. (3).

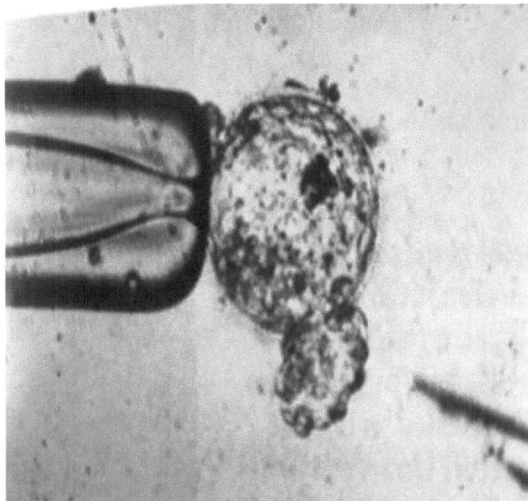

Fig. (3). One of the first ever images of a hatching human blastocyst, taken by the author, at Bourn Hall Clinic in the early 1980's. The embryo is held on a glass holding pipette (left) and a micro-knife (right) is approaching to biopsy the embryo.

We also knew however that such a use of human embryos would be highly controversial from a legal, ethical, religious, moral, technical and regulatory viewpoint. Our main concern focussed around the fact that to obtain human embryonic stem cells from a human embryo requires the destruction of a human embryo which is of course destruction of a potential human life. This is a powerful and emotional debate and not one which we as scientists really had the insight or knowledge to resolve despite long and complex discussions with everyone from scientific colleagues to the Pope.

In terms of human embryonic stem cells the discussions really began in earnest in 1998 when James Thomson and his team in the USA announced the creation of the first human embryonic stem cells in the laboratory. This discovery led to fierce scientific debate, lots of media hype and politicians, theologians and medical ethicists joining the fray. Exciting times for stem cells!

The considerable noise and media interested created by the discovery of human embryonic stem cells did not deter other researchers from seeking out stem cells from other tissues in the body. Since we now knew about both mouse and human embryonic stem cells (known generally as embryonic stem cells) the other tissue-based stem cells such as bone marrow became known as adult stem cells. Those stem cells derived from a pregnancy such as cord blood became known as fetal stem cells. It is possible that you have seen the word 'fetal' spelt as 'foetal'. Everyone now accepts that the correct spelling is 'fetal'.

Adult or Fetal Stem Cells?

Bone marrow is clearly an adult stem cell derived from the bone marrow of adult humans. Cord blood stem cells however are placed in the fetal stem cell category because they behave, in some ways, like bone marrow stem cells but are derived from the blood remaining when a baby is born. Cord blood stem cells have other significant differences from adult bone marrow stem cells which will be described further in Chapter 3. There then followed an amazing sequence of events which led to the discovery of many adult and fetal stem cells in a whole range of tissues in the human body which created a lot of hope for some people but unfortunately also a lot of hype for others.

Umbilical Cord Tissue and Placental Tissue Stem Cells

Discoveries were made in 2005 by Dr. John E. Davies (Jed to his friends) and colleagues in Toronto, Canada showing the presence of fetal stem cells (derived from tissue associated with the fetus/baby) in the umbilical cord tissue itself (this is now known as cord tissue). At about the same time fetal 'tissue forming' stem cells were found in the placenta by Dr. B.L.Yen and colleagues in Taiwan.

These two tissues are of course by products of birth (associated with the baby) so it was not long before cord tissue was collected at the same time as cord blood by private cord blood banks as it is relatively easy to cut and save a piece of cord tissue. The stem cells found in cord tissue were found to be 'tissue forming' stem cells which can produce bone, nerve and connective tissue. This discovery provided a new product and a new income stream to private cord blood banks. These cord 'tissue forming' stem cells still however need to be fully understood and characterised before they can be used to treat anyone. The storage of cord tissue stem cells in private cord blood banks is therefore not necessarily a useful product in terms of future treatment until much more research has been completed. Despite this over 90% of private cord blood clients now also store cord tissue.

The placenta, however, is a bigger challenge (literally) because it is a complex organ about the size of a dinner plate and about 2-3cm in thickness and is therefore much more difficult to collect process and store. The placenta provides nutrients and oxygen to the baby during development and also removes waste products from the baby. Due to the large size and complexity of this organ the use of placental stem cells in the development of potential treatments lags behind those derived from cord tissue. Research is needed to develop an easy and reliable method of collection and processing the human placenta.

The stem cells discovered in cord tissue and placenta have very different properties to those found in bone marrow and cord blood which are 'blood forming'. The stem cells in placenta and cord tissue are fetal stem cells (derived from the fetus/baby or the tissues associated with the fetus/baby) but they can produce adult connective tissue such a tendons, cartilage, bone, fat and nerves.

These 'tissue forming' stem cells were first discovered in 1976 as a second type of stem cell in bone marrow by Alexander Friedenstein and colleagues. There were found to be very few 'tissue forming' stem cells in the bone marrow and no one really understood their significance. The discovery of umbilical cord tissue and placenta 'tissue forming' fetal stem cells led to the proposal of their potential use in the treatment and repair of tendons and spinal discs, treatment of muscular diseases and trauma and bone disorders such as osteoarthritis. This was the first time when there was a source of easily accessible 'tissue forming' stem cells which could be collected, processed and frozen for later use to treat a wide range of diseases. Regenerative medicine, or at least the basic concept of regenerative medicine, was born!

Fat Stem Cells!

Dr P.A. Zuk and her colleagues in the USA in 2002 took the next important step in the discovery of stem cell types when they reported the presence of stem cells in adipose tissue or fat. The mechanical processing of adipose stem cells from human fat can be seen in Fig. (**4**). The small Lipocube SVF box contains sets of blades which break up the fat as it is passed through the cube by the syringes. This is a very quick and easy method to process fat to obatin adipose stem cells.

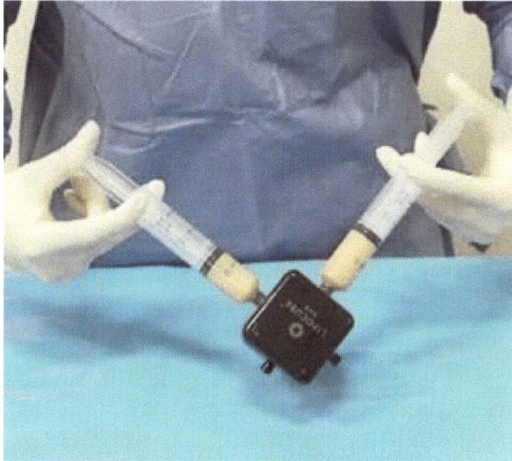

Fig. (4). Human fat (adipose tissue) being processed using a Lipocube mechanical digestion device to produce 'tissue forming' stem cells for treatment.

We all carry around various amounts of fat (some more than others!) but the fact that fat contains stem cells with similar 'tissue forming' properties to cord tissue and placenta means that we are all carrying around a supply of tissue forming stem cells which can be easily harvested as and when needed. The only drawback on this is that as we age then our stem cells also age so harvesting fat at an old age might not be as good as harvesting fat from a young person. Fat stem cells are of course adult stem cells because they are derived from adult tissue and the *potential* of these cells to treat a whole range of diseases in the future is enormous but this story is for Chapter 8.

The Tooth Fairy and Stem Cells

Stem cells then appeared to be everywhere we looked, even inside teeth! In 2005 Dr I Kerkis and her colleagues in Brazil discovered the presence of 'tissue forming' stem cells inside adult teeth and also inside baby teeth. The tooth fairy was furious.

The concept here is that when a healthy adult tooth is extracted for orthodontic reasons, or perhaps an impacted wisdom tooth, then these teeth can be taken to a lab, broken open and the valuable stem cells inside removed and frozen for later use. The same applies when a child loses a 'baby tooth'. Decayed teeth are unfortunately not a good source of stem cells.

There is, to this day, a constant search for new sources of stem cells in all of the tissues of the body and this is not only to seek out potential sources of stem cells for treatments in the future but also to understand the biology of these stem cells to increase our knowledge and understanding of the mechanisms by which stem cells keep us all alive on a daily basis.

'Man Made' Stem Cells

The next step in the evolution of stem cell technology took many of us by surprise. This was because this next discovery moved away from simply seeking out stem cells in different tissues in the body to actually making stem cells on demand from normal body cells. This extraordinary piece of work was carried out in 2006 by Professor Shinya Yamanaka in Japan and Professor Sir John Gurdon in Cambridge. They took normal skin cells and introduced 4 new genes (pieces of genetic information) into these skin cells and then watched what happened. To their great surprise these normal skin cells went 'back in time' to become pluripotent stem cells (stem cells capable of producing nearly every cell type in the body) very similar to human embryonic stem cells. This was a major breakthrough in stem cell technology and both Yamanaka and Gurdon were awarded the Nobel prize in 2012 for their efforts.

The significance of this work is that it is now possible to obtain stem cells, capable of forming all tissue or cell types, from the normal cells of any person completely on demand. There is still much work to be done on these 'man made' stem cells but the excitement in the stem cell community was tremendous and many workers are exploring these opportunities to the present day. These 'man made' stem cells have recently opened the door to the possibility of creating human eggs and sperm in the laboratory and using these 'man made' human gametes to create an IVF baby. Such technology raises many medical, legal, ethical and moral issues but it is an area which all budding stem cell scientists and potential fertility patients should be aware. An additional application of 'man made' stem cells is to use them as the starting point for 'organoids'. Organoids are tiny versions of larger organs such as brain, kidney and liver and enable scientists to study normal organ function, disease processes and pharmaceutical testing in the laboratory. Organoids have considerable potential but there is still a lot to be done to understand if organoids truly represent full size organs and can be reliably used as a model for full size organs.

INITIAL CONCLUSIONS

There are some important messages to take from this Chapter and perhaps the most important is that stem cell technology is nothing new. Stem cell technology has been around since 1956 and we all *still have an enormous amount to learn* about stem cells. The developments in stem cell science since the early days of the first bone marrow transplant have brought the technology out of the laboratory and into the remit of newspapers, the media (including electronic social media), politicians, patients and their families, theologians, business-men and perhaps most worrying some stem cell charlatans. These are people around the globe who promote stem cell technology as a modern day 'snake oil'. They offer untested, unproven and potentially unsafe 'treatments' for every disease under the Sun, to vulnerable or terminally ill patients. Such potential patients must be made aware of the risks and likely effectiveness of such proposed 'treatments' but sadly this is not always the case. The increased level of stem cell awareness brings hopes and fears for patients and Pound or Dollar signs in the eyes of others. Exploitation of vulnerable patients by uncaring, unprofessional, unethical profit driven 'stem cell clinics' must stop.

The following chapters will explore these issues to develop a clear insight into the fascinating and often frustrating subject of Regenerative Medicine and to reflect on the truth, and sometimes the hard reality and hype of the Regeneration Promise.

KEY POINTS OF CHAPTER 1

- Stem cell treatment is nothing new; the first bone marrow transplant dates back to 1956.
- Stem cells are essential for normal health and if and when they go wrong the result can be very serious life-threatening disease.
- Bone marrow stem cell transplantation resulted in an understanding of the importance of tissue matching in transplantation.
- Bone marrow stem cell can today be collected from the blood inside veins, which makes the donation process less invasive.
- Many other stem cells have been discovered since bone marrow stem cells but bone marrow stem cells and cord blood stem cells remain as the *only* source of stem cells in current routine clinical use to treat blood disorders.
- Embryonic stem cells have considerable promise but the practicalities of using them will most likely restrict their use in the future.
- Stem cells from adipose tissue, umbilical cord tissue, placenta, teeth and others

are showing great promise but are not yet in routine clinical use.

• Man-made induced pluripotent stem cells (iPSC) can be used to develop mini organs called organoids, which could be useful in understanding disease processes and developing treatments.

• Great caution is needed by potential patients who are considering stem cell therapy from a private company for a wide range of diseases. These 'treatments' are offered at a very high cost and are often unlicensed operations. Much of these 'treatments' are untested for safety and the effectiveness of the 'treatment' is unknown. Never take part in such 'treatments' they are pointless and might even be dangerous.

CHAPTER 2

Blood and Toil

(Bone marrow transplantation and other applications of bone marrow stem cells)

I have nothing to offer but blood, toil, sweat and tears.
Winston Churchill

Summary: In this chapter, you will learn about the amazing work done with bone marrow transplants to treat leukaemia and blood disorders. This is not an easy process for either the patient or the healthcare professional, but it is a tried and tested treatment for otherwise deadly diseases. There is also a discussion about the nature and importance of clinical trials using bone marrow stem cells to treat a whole range of disease, which is followed by a note of caution to anyone considering such treatment provided by some private clinics outside of registered clinical trials and in areas of the World where regulation of such technology is either weak or non-existent.

'BLOOD FORMING' STEM CELLS

Prior to 1956, the diagnosis of leukaemia and related blood disorders meant that the only outlook was a long, slow, painful death. Once bone marrow transplantation became routine in the 1970's, then effective treatment was a reality. Nevertheless, the treatment process was still technically challenging and not a simple procedure either for the bone marrow donor or the recipient patient.

Before I go any further with this important discussion about bone marrow stem cells, I would like to make one important point very clearly:

'Blood forming' stem cells (whether obtained from bone marrow or *via* peripheral blood or 'blood forming' stem cells from cord blood) are the **only** stem cells in routine clinical use to date and bone marrow stem cells (which includes peripheral blood stem cells) are considered the gold standard for the treatment of blood diseases.

This is extremely important because it clearly emphasises the current and future clinical importance of 'blood forming' stem cells from bone marrow. It also strongly refutes any unproven, untested and unsafe 'treatments' offered by 'clinics' around the World.

There are many Centres of Excellence around the World carrying out 'blood forming' stem cell transplants. Any patient who has to undergo 'blood forming' stem cell transplantation to treat a blood disorder such as leukaemia can be assured that the process is as safe as it can be and that it is supported by considerable amounts of expertise and medical evidence. This medical evidence, usually obtained from papers published in respected medical journals, is known as the evidence base. Stem cell 'clinics' offering untested and unproven 'treatments' almost always have no evidence base or an evidence base, which is either controversial or simply untrue.

The fact that 'blood forming' stem cells are *only* tried and tested in the treatment of blood disorders is extremely important, especially in the light of claims by some companies that bone marrow and/or cord blood stem cells can treat a wide range of diseases unrelated to blood diseases. These claims, without exception, are **all** false or at best based on poor, contradictory, weak or non-existent evidence. When examined closely, it is clear that bone marrow based 'therapies' of this sort are based on hype and untested ideas, and at best can only be supported by incomplete or ongoing clinical trials, which is the way in which such concepts are tested and validated for routine use. The fact that a clinical trial is underway *does not* mean that the safety and efficacy of the subject of the clinical trial are in any way proven. It is only proven if and when the clinical trial is complete and the data show that the subject or treatment being tested proved useful and safe. Even at that point, there could then be many years before the technology in any clinical trial comes into safe routine use. The basic point is that if something is in clinical trial, then it is unproven until it is proven!

There are many workers carrying out research into bone marrow stem cells and creating some interesting and possibly useful information. However, these ideas are *research* and nowhere near clinical application. Such ideas must not be referred to as 'evidence' for clinical use especially by unregulated 'for profit' clinics. They are all interesting examples of basic laboratory research, which may lead to clinical applications in the future. Jumping from basic laboratory research to clinical applications, without clear data on safety and efficacy from *completed* clinical trials which showed a clear benefit, is an extremely dangerous process. It is, however, a very tempting proposition for people who want to make money from vulnerable patients using untested technology.

The only source of 'blood forming' stem cells which even comes close to bone marrow in terms of clinical importance is cord blood. This technology will be explained in detail in Chapter 3. This is therefore, the first big surprise in the Regeneration Promise, which may give the impression that we are routinely using stem cells left, right and centre to treat a whole range of diseases: ***We are not***.

The truth is that bone marrow stem cells (remember these are 'blood forming' stem cells) are routinely used to treat leukaemia and blood disorders, which amount to about 80 different blood diseases when you take into account the various types of leukaemia and genetic disorders which affect the blood system. This makes bone marrow stem cells, *without any doubt*, the most important stem cells in routine clinical use and the basis of all of the subsequent ideas on regenerative medicine and stem cell technology.

Bone Marrow Transplantation

In order to put the clinical use of bone marrow transplantation into perspective and to understand that even bone marrow stem cells are not a perfect or easy option, it is useful to better understand the transplantation process.

The first step in a bone marrow transplant is the initial diagnosis of disease in the recipient patient. In terms of leukaemia this would involve initial blood tests and then taking a small amount of bone marrow, usually from the breast bone under a local anaesthetic, and examining this under a microscope to work out which type of leukaemia or other blood disorder is present. Other genetic blood diseases, such as sickle cell anaemia and thalassaemia can be diagnosed using standard blood tests.

Once we have the diagnosis then the second step is to find a suitable matched bone marrow stem cell donor. This can be a difficult process for some patients. The first stop in this search for a bone marrow donor is usually family members, but surprisingly, this is often unsuccessful unless identical twins are involved, which, as mentioned earlier, are a perfect match for each other. More recently, however, family members have started to be used as donors for 'haploidentical' bone marrow transplantation.

The problem with finding a bone marrow donor is that the donor and recipient must ideally be a 99-100% tissue match. Any bone marrow where the tissue match is less than 99-100% is likely to cause major, potentially fatal GvHD (rejection) complications in the recipient patient. Few transplant physicians will take the risk of using poorly tissue matched donor bone marrow as the outcome for the recipient patients has been shown to be very poor.

Haploidentical Transplantation

More recently, family members have started to be used as donors for 'haploidentical' bone marrow transplantation. When carrying out haploidentical transplantation, it is possible to use medication, which reduce the recipients' immune system reactions in slightly unmatched bone marrow and this proves useful for some patients. This is the basis of haploidentical transplantation. The slightly unmatched haploidentical donor marrow can also have the immune cells, which mediate rejection, removed or depleted. This also results in a better acceptance of the haploidentical bone marrow. As the technology of haploidentical transplantation has improved over recent years, the technique has now become the most common treatment route for blood disorders.

Find the Match

Despite all of this some patients who need a bone marrow transplant still cannot find a suitable donor (even an haploidentical donor) and may even die before a suitable donor can be found. This is especially common when the recipient patient is of mixed race where a suitable match can be very difficult to find. An example of this can be found in Toronto Canada, where there was a mass immigration of Chinese people when Hong Kong was returned to China by the UK. These Chinese people naturally soon found partners in Canada, which often were Caucasian. The tissue type of the resulting children is a complex mix of Asian and Caucasian and resulted in some children in Toronto suffering from blood disorders but unfortunately, with no hope of finding a suitable stem cell donor. This in no way criticises mixed race relationships, it is offered to simply explain the complexity of some tissue typing scenarios, which may result from mixed race relationships. It is up to stem cell scientists to resolve the problem!

Bone Marrow Stem Cell Banks

There are many bone marrow stem cell banks around the world where bone marrow (including peripheral blood stem cells) has been collected from donors, tissue typed and frozen ready for use when needed. Such banks provide databases of the tissue types they hold, which can be searched by physicians looking for a match for their patients. These bone marrow donations are stored in blood bags in liquid nitrogen, under strict monitoring and quality regulations, where they will be stable for many years in storage. When cells are stored in liquid nitrogen (at -196°C) all biological activity stops allowing long term storage (many decades at least) if needed.

These stem cell banks are at the heart of validated, safe and effective 'blood forming' stem cell transplantation for blood disorders.

Preparation for Transplant

Assuming that we find a suitable match for the recipient patient then the next step is to prepare the recipient patient for the transplant, this is called conditioning. This conditioning is the start of a very tough time for the recipient patient and can even be the cause of death in some recipient patients. The reason for this is that the next stage requires the destruction of the diseased bone marrow using chemotherapy (toxic medication) and radiotherapy (X ray treatment). The purpose is to destroy the diseased bone marrow in the recipient patient but the chemotherapy and radiotherapy also effects the rest of the body which will result in the classic hair loss seen in transplant patients and damage to other organs which is not as visible but can be extremely painful and even fatal. As the diseased bone marrow in the recipient patient is destroyed the recipient patient will totally lose their immune system, which protects them from infection, making any opportunistic minor infection potentially fatal. For this reason, bone marrow transplant patients are kept in isolation, in a very controlled clean air atmosphere, to minimise the risk of infection. This isolation will be needed for several months after the transplant before the donor stem cells find their way to the recipient patient bone marrow and get to work to produce new blood cells.

Transplant Time

Once the diseased recipient patient bone marrow has been destroyed then the next step is to prepare the donor bone marrow for transplantation. The frozen donor bone marrow may be easily transported around the World if needed and sent to the hospital treating the recipient. The recipient has a 'central line' inserted which give access to a major blood vessel in the body into which the donor bone marrow is infused. When everyone is satisfied that the diseased bone marrow has been destroyed then the donor bone marrow is thawed and infused into the recipient patient through the central line. This process takes about an hour or so and then the recovery begins!

Recovery

Recovery following bone marrow transplantation is a slow, sometimes painful process, which can take many months. It is also important to remember that this recovery process is all in isolation to prevent infections before the patient has a re-formed an immune system. This can be very tough on the recipient patient both from a medical and a psychological point of view and is an even greater challenge when the recipient patient is a child. Despite this, the transplant teams today are very skilled and experienced and support the patient throughout these difficult times. If all goes well the donated bone marrow stem cells will find the recipient patient bone marrow and will start making new red cells, white cells and platelets and the disease will be gone.

It's Not Easy!

The reason for describing the bone marrow transplant process in some detail is to develop a better understanding about this pioneering use of stem cells in the treatment of blood disorders and to see that stem cell therapy, at least for the blood disorders, is not an 'easy' process. The success rate of bone marrow transplantation for leukaemia and other blood disorders is around 70-80% with deaths resulting most commonly from rejection, bleeding, infection and problems arising from the conditioning regime which in itself is toxic. The patients who need such treatment have little choice but to take these risks associated with transplantation as the alternative is certain death. This makes the risk *versus* benefit of a bone marrow transplant acceptable. This risk is high but the benefit is a subsequent long, healthy life.

'TISSUE FORMING' STEM CELLS IN BONE MARROW

The bone marrow stem cell story does not however stop here. In Chapter 1, I mentioned that bone marrow has also been found to contain 'tissue forming' stem cells. This observation has stimulated researchers to investigate the properties of bone marrow in the treatment of various diseases which brings us nicely back to the Regeneration Promise. In order to properly discuss this next step in bone marrow stem cell discovery and use it is necessary to briefly explain a process called clinical trial and how it relates to discoveries and application in stem cell technology.

Clinical Trials

The concept of a clinical trial has been developed in clinical research to properly assess new medical technology or medication by giving the treatment to a group of human volunteers and seeing if it is of any benefit to those volunteers. It is basically a highly regulated and controlled experiment using human volunteers. The Covid19 pandemic in 2020 highlighted the importance of clinical trials to develop new vaccines and medication or to assess other potential stem cell interventions to treat the severe symptoms of Covid19.

The volunteers in a clinical trial could be fit and healthy people or if the treatment to be tested is for specific disease (*e.g.* Covid19), then volunteers would be patients suffering from that disease.

The next step is to split the volunteers randomly into 2 groups. One of the groups will receive the treatment or medication under investigation and the second group will receive a placebo which is a totally inactive substitute for the medication or treatment. If a placebo is not possible then the placebo group can receive the current approved treatment and comparisons are then made to the medication or treatment being assessed with the current approved treatment. Neither the patients, nor the people carrying out the clinical trial, should know which patients receive the medication or treatment and which patients receive the placebo (or standard treatment) so that all bias is removed. Both groups of patients in the trial are carefully monitored and the results provide information on whether the proposed medication or treatment is beneficial or whether it has no benefit and shows similar results to the placebo or standard treatment group.

Four Phases

Clinical trials are divided into 4 phases which are followed carefully to ensure the results can be confidently relied upon.

- Phase I assesses the safety of the treatment or medication under investigation and it usually involves 10 or less volunteers and no placebo is used in Phase I. If any serious side effects or toxicity is found then the trial would stop at this stage.
- Phase II is when the treatment or medication is tested on usually about 100 further volunteers and some volunteers receive the placebo or standard treatment. Phase II therefore is the first assessment of the efficacy or beneficial action of a new treatment or medication compared to the placebo and also sometimes compared to patients who have received current or 'standard' treatment. Once again if no benefit is found for the new treatment then the clinical trial would stop at phase II. If a benefit is seen at Phase II then the trial goes on to Phase III.
- Phase III involves as many volunteers and treatment centres around the World as possible and is a thorough assessment of the new medication or treatment and will create medical statistics which can clearly prove benefit if it is present.
- Phase IV is the long-term monitoring of the new treatment or medication which is important where side effects may be delayed for months, and even years, after the treatment. Once all phases of the clinical trial are complete and show benefit then the treatment or medication is introduced into routine practice. Clinical trials are therefore very important because they prove the safety and effectiveness of a new treatment or medication and they are considered to be the gold standard in modern clinical research.

I must apologise for that rather large diversion into clinical trials but it is essential to understand clinical trials in the context of the Regeneration Promise. Now that the concept of clinical trial is in mind I can return to the interesting stuff!

BONE MARROW STEM CELLS AND HEART ATTACK

To get back to my much more relevant stem cell story the next step in bone marrow stem cell technology was to start to assess the properties of the 'tissue forming' stem cells which had been found in bone marrow. An application of bone marrow 'tissue forming' cells which created much hope was the idea that these bone marrow 'tissue forming' stem cells would help patients who had suffered a heart attack (known medically as a myocardial infarction or M.I.) to recover better and faster.

The concept here was that the bone marrow stem cells would 'repair' the damaged heart and many cardiologists quickly jumped onto the idea without any real critical thought. The proposal was that when someone has a heart attack then a small sample of bone marrow would be taken from the heart attack patient and given back to that same patient (known as an autologous transplant) by directly injecting it into the heart at the site of damage to the heart. Before you worry about a massive needle being plunged into the chest of a feeble heart attack victim let me reassure you that the bone marrow stem cells were delivered by cardiac catheter *via* an artery in the wrist or the groin in the same way that a stent is delivered to the coronary arteries. This is nevertheless an invasive procedure with the risks of bleeding or infection.

The next step in this seemingly great idea was to move to clinical trial and Phase I seemed to show no safety issues but no clear benefits so Phase II quickly followed. Then the problems started. The patients who received bone marrow did no better than those who received standard treatment (a placebo was not used as it would be unethical to treat a potentially fatal heart attack with a placebo!). Some people tried to claim that benefits were still seen but it soon became clear that this particular application of bone marrow 'tissue forming' stem cells was hype over hope and the trials stopped. When these patients were followed up, following death, it was found that no bone marrow stem cells were still present in the heart and there was no sign at all of any 'repair' of the tissue damaged during the heart attack.

There were several problems with these stem cell ideas not least the assumption that bone marrow 'tissue forming' stem cells were present in sufficient numbers and could somehow repair damaged heart tissue. It is of course easy to criticise with hindsight but in this case the momentum and enthusiasm seemed to get the better of everyone. Just logical thinking can see that a 'blood forming' stem cell, with the best will in the world, cannot repair heart muscle. There was, in fact, *no evidence at all* for the potential of bone marrow stem cells to repair heart tissue but the trials still went ahead. The Emperors' new clothes were once again not up to standard!

Some may think that this is of course easy to say with hindsight but as you will see later in this book these assumptions are still made too often by some scientists, and many ill-advised profit greedy business men, and the results can be very damaging to the patient and very expensive. Caution is needed at all stages and everything must be evidence based (based on the science) and not based on hope, hype, wishful thinking or a clinical trial which is underway but has yet to produce any data. The basic message here is that the wrong stem cell for the job was chosen and the outcome was, not suprisingly, totally negative. It also highlights an important point that it is essential to use the right stem cell for the right job to achieve the Regeneration Promise.

BONE MARROW STEM CELLS AND AUTOIMMUNE DISEASE

There has been a lot of good work recently on the concept of using bone marrow stem cell transplantation to treat autoimmune disease such as multiple sclerosis. An autoimmune disease occurs when the bodies' immune system goes wrong and starts to recognise normal body cells as foreign and in turn to destroy them. In diseases such as multiple sclerosis the patients' own immune system start to attack nerve cells in the brain and the resulting symptoms can be extremely serious. Multiple sclerosis in known to be a relapsing/remitting disease which means that people suffering from multiple sclerosis may have periods when they are well and periods when the disease and symptoms return.

The concept of using bone marrow stem cell to treat multiple sclerosis is very interesting and could help some patients. The process is as follows:

• The patient receives medication to mobilise bone marrow stem cells into the blood and these are collected using apheresis as described in Chapter 5
• The stem cells are then frozen and the patient then undergoes chemotherapy to destroy their existing immune system
• Once the chemotherapy is complete then the frozen stem cells are thawed and given back to the patient

The theory here is that this process 're-boots' the patients' immune system to bring it back to normal function so that the immune cells no longer attack the brain and symptoms should subside. The process will not repair any existing damage in the brain but it may stop any further damage.

This procedure has strict eligibility criteria such as age and extent of the disease. A patient with advanced relapsing MS is unlikely to be offered bone marrow stem cell transplantation as a treatment option whereas a young, recently diagnosed patient with long remission periods may fare well from a bone marrow stem cell transplant.

The procedure is available in most countries now and it is approved and funded by the NHS in the UK.

There are of course risks to such a bone marrow transplant to treat multiple sclerosis which have been described earlier in this Chapter. As in most areas of medicine physicians have to assess the risk of a procedure against the possible benefits. If this risk to benefit ratio appears to be acceptable then bone marrow transplantation may be offered to these patients and the outcome can be very beneficial to the patient suffering from multiple sclerosis.

This is a relatively new procedure so at present we do not really know if the immune system "re-boot" is permanent but the data so far look promising.

THE RIGHT STEM CELL AND A HOLISTIC APPROACH

The idea of the right stem cell for the right job is very important in regenerative medicine. It is analogous to ensuring that the right standard medication is used for the right disease symptoms.

For example, if you have a headache then you take some painkillers and not an asthma medication! The exact same principle applies to stem cell therapy: If you have a damaged bone then the stem cell used to try to repair this damage must be known to be capable of producing bone and this must be documented in the medical literature as doing so.

This is, of course, common sense but some people in the stem cell industry do not seem to have any common sense.

At present it is possible that we may be expecting too much from stem cells and trying to use them in situations where they are either wrong for the job or are simply destroyed in the diseased target tissue by an angry, destructive environment. Some 'tissue forming' stem cells have been given intravenously in attempts to resolve disease in specific organs or tissue. This is a very big ask for two reasons:

1. If 'tissue forming' stem cells are given intravenously then the size of the stem cell means that they will get caught in the lungs and go no further

2. If 'tissue forming' stem cells do find their way to the place where they are needed then in advanced disease it is unlikely that they can have much impact on their own

This is an area of active research where there is still much for us to learn and this knowledge will refine and improve stem cell therapies.

Another point which must be made is that at present some people are expecting too much from stem cell therapy *alone*. Stem cells are *not magic* and they cannot be expected to cure everything on their own. The idea that an injection of stem cells alone will cure or stop a disease is at best niave and at worst incompetent or reckless. Even the very successful bone marrow transplantation relies on not only stem cells but also on a considerable amount of medication, therapy and post-transplant care to be a success. If a stem cell therapy is used then it must be used in a holistic way if the benefits are to be optimised. For example, the patient may need supplements (known scientifically as nutraceuticals) as part of therapy and may need other interventions such as standard medication, lifestyle changes, weight loss or weight gain, physiotherapy and psychological support in order to achieve the desired result. The patient may also need multiple sessions of this holistic stem cell therapy before a benefit is seen. Stem cell therapy, especially that related to regenerative medicine, is not a 'one-shot wonder' and anyone who claims this is sadly misled or seeks to mislead. If the stem cell therapy is to work then it is also not unreasonable to expect that 'booster' treatments will be needed in the future in order to maintain the benefits to the patient. This is not failure, this is nature and we have to work with it, not against it. The combination of stem cells and other technology and support strategies are needed in a given treatment strategy for success. At present not many, if any, people in regenerative medicine work to this principle which will eventually give stem cell therapy a bad reputation as the overall results of stem cell therapy appear negative because of poor practice. If we can take a holistic approach, allowing bone marrow transplantation to be our model, then stem cell therapy in the future will grow and succeed.

BONE MARROW STEM CELLS AND OSTEOARTHRITIS

Bearing in mind the right stem cell for the right job, a second and possibly more effective use of bone marrow 'tissue forming' stem cells is in the treatment of joint disease such as osteoarthritis. The principle here is that the bone marrow 'tissue forming' stem cells will repair the damaged linings inside the joints and therefore be a significant benefit to patients suffering from osteoarthritis. This is a sensible proposition because the stem cells in this case are known to be capable of doing the job required as the 'tissue forming' stem cells in bone marrow are known to be capable of producing bone and connective tissue which is exactly what is damaged in osteoarthritis. The main concern with this proposal is that the stem cells will be placed into a highly inflamed area (an osteoarthritic joint) and such a place is potentially deadly to the stem cells being used. Nevertheless, 'tissue forming' stem cells are known to be capable of reducing the inflammatory response so in this case we might have the right cell for the right job.

Several workers and clinics have reported success in using bone marrow 'tissue forming' stem cells in the treatment of osteoarthritis but once again the stem cells cannot do it alone so careful attention to standard medication where needed and support such as physiotherapy must be part of the overall treatment package.

Clinical Trials

At the time of writing, there were 11 clinical trials (either recruiting or completed) using bone marrow 'tissue forming' stem cells (derived from the patient being treated) to treat osteoarthritis. The results so far are very encouraging with many patients showing a reduction in disease and pain and in increased mobility in the treated joint. These results *do not* mean that bone marrow 'tissue forming' stem cells are anywhere near being the standard treatment for osteoarthritis and anyone thinking about getting involved in such a treatment must view it as a clinical trial and not a tried and tested safe treatment. Please *take independent unbiased advice* from the physician treating you if you are considering such a treatment. The technology may one day become part of routine clinical practice but this will take many more studies and confirmation of the safety and effectiveness of the treatment which will take several years. It is also very important to note that participation in a clinical trial does not cost the patient anything and indeed in many clinical trials the patient actually receives payment for volunteering. If you consider becoming a volunteer in a clinical trial please make sure that you understand your roles and responsibilities before agreeing to any involvement and ensure that you receive and give informed consent to take part in the clinical trial.

BONE MARROW AND OTHER DISEASES

In addition to these clinical trials using bone marrow 'tissue forming' stem cells there are at the time of writing 167 clinical trials recruiting volunteers using bone marrow 'tissue forming' stem cells to treat a wide range of diseases such as autism, neurodegenerative disease (for example amyotrophic lateral sclerosis or Lou Gehring's disease) and even spinal cord injury. Once again, these clinical trials *do not* mean that any of these applications are tried and tested, it merely means that work is underway to properly assess the possibilities and that routine treatments *may* result in the future if the results support the concept. If anyone tries to tell you that these applications are in clinical trial and therefore can be offered for routine treatment (especially for a large fee) then they are deliberately seeking to mis-lead and they should be reported to the relevant authorities. The problem here of course is that some Countries do not have any stem cell regulation authorities.

This discussion about clinical trials may seem a little academic but it illustrates a very important point that, apart from the treatment of leukaemia, blood disorders and in some cases multiple sclerosis (using the autologous transplantation immune system 're-boot' concept), bone marrow stem cells ('blood forming' or 'tissue forming') are *not at present in proven routine clinical practice for any other applications*. This means that any offers you may see using any type of bone marrow stem cell to treat anything (apart from leukaemia, blood disorders and in some circumstances multiple sclerosis) is being offered with often questionable or non-existent evidence of the safety and effectiveness of the treatment. Equally such treatments should not be offered by companies for profit (for a fee) and the advertising of such treatments should be restricted by regulatory authorities to avoid exploitation of vulnerable patients. If you are offered bone marrow stem cell treatment by a company asking any fee for the service then please either decline or refer to the advice given in Chapter 11 of this book. This will ensure your safety and wellbeing in the sometimes murky world of the Regeneration Promise.

KEY POINTS OF CHAPTER 2

- Bone marrow or 'blood forming' stem cells from bone marrow, peripheral blood or cord blood are the **only** stem cells in routine clinical practice to treat blood disease.
- The diagnosis, donation and transplantation of bone marrow stem cells is a highly technical and demanding process, especially for the stem cell recipient.
- Bone marrow 'tissue forming' stem cells were assessed as a possible treatment of heart attack, but the clinical trials showed that the technology was ineffective.
- Bone marrow 'tissue forming' stem cells may have potential in the treatment of some diseases such as osteoarthritis, but they are not yet fully understood and these are all in clinical trial only.
- Bone marrow stem cell transplantation is used in some cases to 're-boot' the immune system in patients suffering from multiple sclerosis.
- Companies offering a wide range of treatments for different diseases using bone marrow stem cells do not have the evidence needed to support their claims. Please avoid such companies for your own health and safety.
- If you are considering receiving a stem cell treatment from a private stem cell company to treat any disease then the best advice is to discuss it with an unbiased physician first. Offers from private stem cell companies are often too

good to be true and draw in vulnerable and frightened patients very easily.

- Tissue forming stem cells are being assessed in many clinical trials around the World but this **does not** mean that this technology is either safe or effective. Much more work is needed and patients offered such treatments are advised to obtain a second unbiased opinion.
- A holistic approach is recommended when using stem cell therapy to maximise the best outcome for each patient.

CHAPTER 3

A Bouncing Baby!

(The introduction of umbilical cord blood stem cell transplantation and CP/autism research)

A baby is like the beginning of all things – wonder, hope, a dream of possibilities.
Eda J. Le Shan

Summary: This chapter provides an introduction to cord blood stem cells and how they can be used in the treatment of leukaemia and blood disorders. The pros and cons of using cord blood stem cells for transplantation are also discussed. It also explores the ground-breaking clinical trials on the use of cord blood to treat cerebral palsy and autism.

CORD BLOOD STEM CELLS

In chapter 2, it was mentioned that cord blood is a useful source of 'blood forming' stem cells which can supplement and sometimes even replace the tried and tested bone marrow stem cells. In this Chapter, I will describe the use of cord blood stem cells, which have now been used to treat over 80 blood disorders, including leukaemia and related blood diseases, since the first transplant in 1988.

When a baby is born anywhere in the World, there is quite rightly great joy for the new life it brings. New parents, grandparents, uncles and aunts all wish the new baby health, wealth and happiness. Foremost of all of those is health and we all wish that all children could remain in good health. Sadly, this is not the case and some children will inevitably go on to develop serious life-threatening diseases such as leukaemia and cancer. Many of these children will die simply because of the lack of a suitable bone marrow donor, as described in earlier chapters. There is a simple and effective solution for some of these children and small adults and this is umbilical cord blood stem cell transplantation.

Cord Blood Stem Cell Collection Process

When a baby is delivered, and the umbilical cord is clamped and cut, there is the blood left in the umbilical cord and placenta. This 'cord blood' contains life giving 'blood-forming' stem cells which could potentially one day save that baby's life, the life of a member of the baby's family or even the life of an unrelated patient. The stem cells found in cord blood are stem cells which are capable of replacing diseased or damaged bone marrow. In the case of the umbilical cord blood, the 'blood forming' stem cells are present in large numbers and they are capable of forming all of the cells of the blood system.

The collection of umbilical cord blood stem cells is very simple. Once the baby has been born, and the umbilical cord has been clamped and cut, it is simply a matter of putting a needle into the umbilical cord and allowing the blood to drain into a specially designed cord blood collection bag. This process, collecting cord blood before delivery of the placenta, is shown in Fig. (5). Most cord blood today is collected after the delivery of the placenta. The process takes no more than 2-5 minutes. The cord blood is collected by a trained phlebotomist and it does not interfere in any way with the birthing process or different birthing practices such as water births. Research and development are underway to optimize this collection process, perhaps using automation, so that the volume and quality of cord blood collected can be maximised, which will in turn, increase the clinical utility of cord blood.

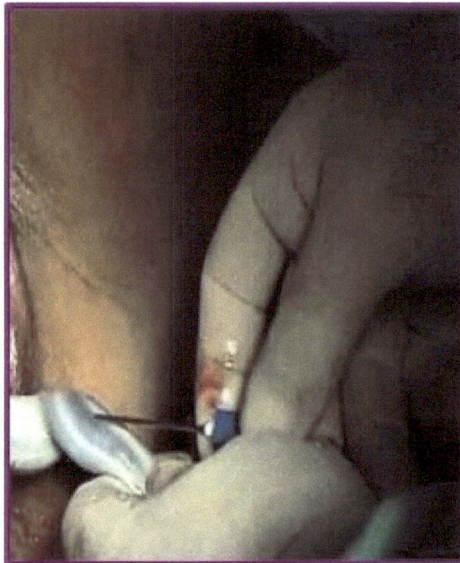

Fig. (5). The collection of umbilical cord blood before delivery of the placenta.

Cord Blood Stem Cell Storage Options

There are commercial companies around the World offering private cord blood collection and storage to pregnant women for a fee (usually between £3000-

5000). The fee covers the collection, processing and first year of storage for the cord blood stem cells and there is an additional annual storage fee (usually about £100 per year). The concept here in these private cord blood banks is that the stored cord blood can be used to treat the baby or a family member (most commonly siblings or parents) if needed. The chance of such cord blood being needed for family use is around 1:1000, so there are many privately stored cord blood stem cells which are never used.

The other option for pregnant women is to donate their cord blood to a public cord blood bank where it will be made available to anyone in need. This does not cost the pregnant mother anything and the chance of using the cord blood is much higher. Nevertheless, if the cord blood stem cells are needed in the family, then there is no guarantee that they will still be available. The subject of private *versus* public cord blood banks is discussed in detail in Chapter 4.

Following collection, the cord blood bag is then placed into a shipping container and sent to the processing laboratory using a medical courier. The cord blood collection bag does not need any special treatment, it is kept at room temperature and the stem cells it contains are stable for up to 72 hours following collection. The collection of umbilical cord blood as described has no effect whatsoever on the baby or the mother.

Cord Blood Laboratory Processing

On arrival at the laboratory, the cord blood collection bag is carefully assessed by carefully trained scientists to ensure that no damage or adverse temperature variations have occurred during transport. The collection kit is designed to provide optimum protection to cord blood during transit to the laboratory. Once accepted and shown to be safe, the cord blood is then processed. The processing is the same for public and private cord blood banks.

The processing most commonly involves the removal of excess plasma and red cells from the cord blood by using the validated technology such as the widely used Sepax system. The volume reduction achieves a concentrated (the total volume is 25mL) solution of the potentially life-giving stem cells in a bag about the same size as a credit card. The cord blood stem cells are then slowly frozen from room temperature to -180°C in a controlled rate freezing machine (such as that produced by Planer) to final storage in liquid nitrogen at -196°C. The liquid nitrogen tanks in which cord blood stem cells (and other stem cell types) are stored have 24/7 monitoring and alarm systems which alert the laboratory staff if the storage temperature goes out of range. The stem cells are completely stable at this very low temperature (biological activity is stopped and kept in suspended animation) and can be stored for many years. Samples of umbilical cord stem cells which have been stored frozen for 15 years have been thawed to assess the quality of the long-term frozen cells. On thawing, they were as good as the day they were frozen. If the cells are needed to treat a disease such as leukaemia or other blood disorders in the baby or a direct relative, and the parents use a private cord blood bank, then the stem cells are released from the private cord blood bank to the physician treating the individual precisely at the time they are needed. The stem cells are released for transplant whilst still frozen making it possible to send the stem cells anywhere in the world for transplant. This process of private cord blood collection and storage means that there is no need to search for a suitable donor, a process which often fails or finds a donor when the disease is too far progressed for treatment.

Cord Blood Stem Cells Pros and Cons

The transplantation process using cord blood stem cells is the same as that for bone marrow or peripheral blood stem cells. There are however, some important practical differences when using cord blood stem cells for transplantation. The most notable of these differences is that cord blood stem cells do not need a 100% tissue match between donor and recipient to be transplanted safely. Indeed, some transplant centres have safely transplanted cord blood stem cells with up to a 50% mismatch between donor and recipient. This is thought to be because cord blood stem cells are fetal stem cells (derived from the birth of a baby) and as such, they are relatively 'undeveloped' from an immunology point of view when compared to adult stem cells from the bone marrow. The proposal is that these 'undeveloped' stem cells are more readily accepted by the immune system of the recipient patient but the actual mechanism is yet to be fully understood.

It has also been found that the donor cord blood stem cells often take longer to become fully operational in the recipient (this is a process called engraftment) following transplant especially in the production of platelets, which are a component of blood, which is involved in blood clotting. This slower engraftment time means that the recipient of a cord blood stem cell transplant may be more susceptible to an infection or bleeding post-transplant than a recipient of bone marrow stem cells. This problem can of course be managed relatively easily by an experienced transplant team by careful monitoring of the patient and by using platelet transfusions if needed.

A final disadvantage when using cord blood stem cells as a transplant is that the cord blood from one cord blood collection only contains enough stem cells to treat a recipient patient who weighs no more than 30 Kg. For this reason, most cord blood transplants have been transplanted to children or small adults.

Perhaps one of the most remarkable examples of a cord blood transplant to a small adult is that of Patrizia Durante in Canada. Patrizia was three months pregnant when she was diagnosed to be suffering from leukaemia and her doctors initially told her that she would die from the leukaemia shortly after the birth of her baby. Patrizia did not accept this and soon found out about cord blood stem cells and how they can treat leukaemia. When her baby was born, the cord blood was collected and subsequently used to treat Patrizia. Patrizia and her baby, Victoria Angel, are alive and well today! This event inspired two colleagues of mine in Toronto, Dr. Mike Virro and his wife Jane, (who together had already set-up Cells For Life which is a very successful private cord blood bank) to set up a public cord blood bank called the Victoria Angel Registry of Hope in Toronto. This public cord blood bank still supplies cord blood stem cells to anyone in need making a critical contribution to cord blood stem cell transplantation in Canada and potentially overseas. It was an honour for me to be involved in the early stages of the development of the Victoria Angel Registry of Hope.

Patrizia was lucky in a way in that she is a relatively small person and when she was ill, there were just enough stem cells in the cord blood collected from her daughter Victoria Angel to regenerate her bone marrow. Had she been physically larger than the story might have been very different.

Cord Blood Stem Cell Double Transplants and Expansion

If the recipient patient is physically too large (greater than 30Kg in weight at the time of transplant) for the number of cord blood stem cells which are available in one cord blood donation (called a cord blood unit), then there are 2 options available to the physicians treating these patients:

- The first option is to use more than one cord blood unit on one patient. Many patients have received double, and even triple, cord blood transplants and, because of the inherent biological 'flexibility' of cord blood stem cells, the stem cells from different donors are able to work together to regenerate the bone marrow of a large adult patient. It is even possible to detect blood cells derived from the different donors in the blood of the recipient patients and there are many patients now in the World with 2 or even 3 different types of donor cells in their bodies.
- The second option is to use a technology known as cell expansion, where one cord blood unit is treated in the laboratory with specific chemicals and growth factors to create enough stem cells from one cord blood unit to treat a patient weighing over 30 Kg. This cell expansion approach has been shown to work in a few clinical trials but there is still a lot of work to do to identify the best expansion technology. This external human manipulation of the cord blood also

introduces some additional regulatory requirements which need to be resolved before such technology can get into routine clinical practice. Once any cell type has been manipulated, it becomes a 'medication' or a 'pharmaceutical' and as such has to meet all of the regulations which apply to pharmaceuticals. The cost and inconvenience of this is the primary barrier to any form of cell expansion being used in routine clinical applications but many researchers are working on this problem.

Quality not Quantity

There has recently been a proposal that stem cell quality and not quantity should be the priority and technology has been proposed, which increases stem cell 'quality'. The quality of a stem cell could be better assessed by technology, which can detect the ability of the stem cell to divide, cell membrane damage, cell surface molecules and components inside the stem cell such as the nucleus and the quality of the DNA it contains. This approach could, in theory, make it possible to transplant fewer higher quality cord blood stem cells than is thought to be needed but to still achieve the desired outcome of engraftment in the recipient patient. These ideas and technology are yet to be fully tested and proven but the concept is interesting and potentially useful. If this approach is proven to be safe and effective, it could extend the use of cord blood stem cells in the treatment of blood disorders and also have a big impact on cellular therapy in general.

Cord Blood Stem Cell Clinical Trial for Cerebral Palsy

Cord blood is clearly a useful option open to physicians when treating blood disorders but other applications not related to blood disorders, are showing some promise. Ongoing clinical trials in the USA (most notably at Duke University led by Dr Joanne Kurtzberg) and other centres are underway to assess if cord blood can potentially be used to treat children suffering from cerebral palsy and autism. These cord blood cells are truly *potential* givers of life not only in blood disorders but also *potentially* in the treatment of neurological disorders. At the time of writing there are 6 clinical trials focussing on the treatment of cerebral palsy and they are using both cord blood collected from the patients themselves (autologous treatment) and also using cord blood collected from other people (allogeneic treatment) to treat the patients. The results so far for cerebral palsy are encouraging, with many patients seeming to benefit from the treatment but much more work is needed before this becomes a routine treatment for cerebral palsy. One of the problems is trying to assess how individual patients would have been without any treatment as the progress of cerebral palsy is quite difficult in any one patient. It is worth adding that these patients do not require any conditioning (chemotherapy and radiation) prior to their cord blood treatment, the cord blood is simply infused into a vein in the same way as a blood transfusion and the clever cord blood cells do the rest. The mechanism of action, including whether or not the cord blood cells actually make it to the brain and if so, what they do there, is at present unknown. The brain in normal health is protected by a 'wall' called the blood-brain barrier. In normal life, this acts to stop unwanted cells, materials and other foreign substances from entering the brain. The blood-brain barrier is not perfect. Many things can cross the blood-brain barrier, such as bacteria and viruses and it can be damaged in disease so that other things also get access to the brain. The size of a cord blood stem cells should prevent them from entering the brain but the benefits seen seem to indicate that in cerebral palsy they might be getting access to the brain. The possible benefit to cerebral palsy patients seen in clinical trials could be from the cord blood stem cells themselves crossing the blood-brain barrier or from chemicals (known as growth factors and cytokines) produced by the cord blood stem cells, which can easily cross the blood-brain barrier and act on nerve cells to repair any damage. At present, we do not know which, if any, of the explanations are correct, but the potential is immense for children suffering from cerebral palsy.

Cord Blood Stem Cell Clinical Trial for Autism

The Phase II clinical trial at Duke University using cord blood stem cells to treat autism has shown in May 2020 that cord blood has no clear beneficial effect on autism patients. This work has been stopped and if it goes back to clinical trial once more, then the technology will have to be very much refined.

Dr Joanne Kurtzberg and her team at Duke University have recently decided to patent their technology relating to the use of cord blood in the treatment of cerebral palsy and autism. The plans to patent the technology related to autism are now on hold because of the negative clinical trial data. Nevertheless, this means that those patients who receive cord blood in the future as a treatment for cerebral palsy will now need to pay for the treatment if this is part of the final patent. This is a sad development in an otherwise exciting technology. Patents, in my opinion, do not really have a place in healthcare because they immediately limit the accessibility of the treatment which has been patented. Nevertheless, commercial pressures often persist and patents are issued on a regular basis both for new technologies and new medications. It is important to note that patents cannot be taken out on anything which exists naturally, for example stem cells. The patent usually covers the technology, perhaps either the preparation of the cells for use or the protocol used for transplantation. Patents are also only valid in certain Countries so for example a patent registered in the USA might not be valid or enforceable in the UK. There can be global patents but these are comparatively rare.

Cord blood stem cells seem to have enormous potential and there are no doubt many more discoveries to be made. Despite this cord, cloud stem cells do have their limitations and it is important to understand these limitations to prevent hype from being stronger than hope. The challenge for the scientists and physicians is to optimize the use of cord blood stem cells and perhaps even bring them into use for diseases that have yet to be thought about. This will be the true Regeneration Promise and only in decades to come will we know the true answers.

KEY POINTS OF CHAPTER 3

- Cord blood 'blood forming' stem cells can be collected at every birth and contain stem cells which can treat blood disorders. They are therefore a useful alternative to bone marrow 'blood forming' stem cells.
- Cord blood can be kept in a private bank for family use only or donated to a public bank for use by anyone in need.
- Cord blood stem cells do not need a 100% tissue match and so can be used more easily than bone marrow stem cells.
- A cord blood collection only contains enough stem cells to treat a patient weighing no more than 30Kg. If the patient is larger then multiple cord blood transplants can be used using cord blood from 2 or more different donors. It is also possible to expand cord blood stem cell numbers in the laboratory which is another treatment option for larger patients.
- Cord blood has shown promise in the treatment of cerebral palsy and advanced clinical trials are underway.
- Cord blood has been shown to be ineffective in initial clinical trials for the treatment of autism.

CHAPTER 4

Baby Blues

(The issues surrounding public and private cord blood storage and use)

We are our choices This is a quote.
Jean-Paul Sartre

Summary: This chapter explores the subject of public and private cord blood collection and storage and tries to answer some of the frequently asked questions about these services. It provides specific advice for those people considering private cord blood banking and explains the pros, cons and practicalities of cord blood collection and storage. Private cord blood collection and storage has become an enormous business on a global scale, but it is extremely important that the clients of these private cord blood banks fully understand the exact uses and limitations of what is on offer. Ultimately private storage is a matter of personal choice and, of course, a matter of having sufficient money to pay for private cord blood storage.

CHOICES

Life is full of choices. Our partners, our home, a car, when and if to have children, the colour scheme for the lounge and even what to eat this evening. Our whole lives, and the relative success of those lives, are based on choices. Bad choices: bad life. Good choices: good life. We all understand this and we all try our very best to make good choices but inevitably, things can go wrong. This is the human condition, we cannot all be right all of the time. Even I might have made some poor choices in the past, but that is a different and scary story!

There is now another choice to add to that list and this is whether or not to collect and store cord blood from the birth of a baby to create a source of stem cells for family if needed. This is perhaps one of the most complex choices asked of parents, at a time when parents (and especially first-time parents) have quite a bit on their minds. The cord blood choice is something for which they are ill prepared, and sometimes ill informed, to make, and this can result in the permanent loss of some of the most precious cells in the world, which have the ability to save a life. Life is all about choices.

The conundrum when thinking about private cord blood collection and storage is that if a choice is made to store cord blood, it might never be needed and if a choice is made to discard cord blood, then there is no second chance unless there is a second baby.

Public and Private Cord Blood Banks

The previous chapter introduced cord blood stem cells and mentioned the existence of private and public cord blood banks. It is now important to explore this subject a little more because cord blood stem cells are present at the birth of every child and there is a clear choice on what to do with this valuable material: collect and store it for future use if needed or burn it with all the medical waste.

First of all, we need some clear definitions:

- Private cord blood banks collect and store cord blood for *family use only* for an initial fee and an ongoing annual storage fee.
- Public cord blood banks collect and store altruistically donated cord blood for use by anyone in need. There is no cost to the cord blood donor.

The pregnant woman and her partner are often therefore faced with several difficult choices regarding the fate of their cord blood:

- Do we pay to store cord blood stem cells privately which will be kept for our family use only and pay a relatively large collection, processing and storage fee and recurrent annual storage fees to do so?
- Do we donate the cord blood to a public bank for general use, which will cost us nothing and could help someone in need?
- Do we simply ignore the issue altogether and allow the cord blood to be discarded along with the placenta and umbilical cord as medical waste?

The answer in part to these questions may be relatively simple if the parents have a low income and simply cannot afford private collection and storage, which costs about £2000 in the UK, about twice as much in the USA and about a quarter as much in India. These prices around the world may, of course, relate to the relative income of clients and also the income of those working in private cord blood banks (which has to be paid by the income produced from clients) in these countries. They also reflect the expensive technology, highly trained staff, complex facilities, licensing and accreditation costs and expensive high-cost consumables used to collect, process and store cord blood. These costs, of course, vary enormously from country to country.

What would be a better approach is if public health providers (for example, the NHS in the UK) or health insurance companies or companies as a perk of employment could fund the private collection, processing and storage of cord blood for *all* pregnant women. It may even be possible to add cord blood to the existing organ donation legislation in the UK, making cord blood collection automatic unless the mother opts out. This is something which politicians need to hear and make decisions. The cost of this to the health care provider would be high, but no higher than other services and the potential benefits would be enormous. The NHS does currently fund some cord blood banking in the UK but it is for public not private use and it is very restricted. This restriction is because cord blood can only be collected in certain hospitals in the UK so that many pregnant women who wish to donate cord blood cannot. There is also no infrastructure in the UK or elsewhere to enable cord blood donation by all pregnant women.

The Development of Private Cord Blood Banking

In the early days of private cord blood stem cell banking in the early 1990's the advertising used by some private cord blood banks was far from ideal in that some would suggest that private cord blood storage should be carried out by parents because it may save the life of their baby. This is wrong at many levels.

Firstly, the chance of the baby him/herself needing the cord blood and the stored cord blood stem cells being suitable for treatment is remote. Several people have tried to estimate this chance and values from 1:10,000 and 1:100,000 have been suggested. It is safe to assume that privately stored cord blood is highly unlikely to be needed by, or used by, the baby. There is also some evidence that some diseases which are seen in the baby could start during early fetal development. If this proves to be the case, and for some diseases the evidence is becoming more and more convincing, then the stem cells from that baby could simply be the source of more disease once transplanted back to the baby. The fact is that most, if not all, babies will have a better outcome in cord blood stem cell transplantation for blood disorders if the stem cells for transplant come from a matched donor rather than from the baby him/herself.

Secondly this type of marketing, where the parents are led to think that their actions could be the difference between life and death for their baby, is totally unacceptable emotional blackmail. Luckily, this type of advertising by private cord blood banks has now been outlawed by the regulatory authorities and private

cord blood banks are now, *in most countries at least*, obliged to use factual material in their marketing with no emotional blackmail.

This use of scientific evidence to support a given procedure or treatment is the concept of 'evidence based' medicine. The evidence is gained from peer reviewed publications in medical journals. This is the foundation of all medical practice and it is unfortunately still not followed by some in the stem cell industry. This results in silly claims about stem cell 'treatments' which are totally untested and unproven and are the fantasy of marketing men.

There are also legal restrictions relating to the collection of cord blood for private storage in some countries such as France where cord blood cannot be collected or processed for private storage. In other countries, such as Italy, private cord blood collection is allowed but the cord blood itself cannot be processed and stored in Italy and is sent overseas, most commonly to the UK, for processing and storage. Other Countries, such as Spain and Portugal, have a strong private cord blood processing and storage industry and the ethos of 'family' is strong making the use of private cord blood stem banking in the family very attractive in these Countries. This information only serves to add further confusion and the important message is that private cord blood storage is for the family, not the baby.

The Development of Public Cord Blood Banking

Many pregnant women would simply prefer to donate their cord blood for use by anyone in need. This altruistic act is to be praised and supported where it can be achieved. The problem here is that the infrastructure in place to enable this donation is limited and excludes most women from donation. In the UK, for example, there are less than 10 maternity units across the whole country where cord blood can be collected for donation. Donation of cord blood is therefore not really an option for most pregnant women and results in the loss of precious cord blood stem cells which could otherwise have saved lives. More resources are needed (mostly money which will translate into increased facilities and staff) in the public cord blood sector to allow this option to be taken up by more women but the public healthcare providers, such as the NHS in the UK, have many other more pressing priorities. Pressure needs to be put on politicians globally to provide better global public cord blood education, collection, processing and storage infrastructure to reduce the needless loss of cord blood stem cells which are a precious life-saving resource. At present 99% of cord blood is discarded globally as medical waste.

Public cord blood banks charge a fee (typically around £10,000 and sometimes more) to the transplant hospital when they release a cord blood unit for transplantation which goes some way to fund the public collection, processing and storage of cord blood. Despite this, cord blood banking is a very expensive process and additional government funding is required in all Countries if a public cord blood bank is to function properly.

The final option is to simply allow the cord blood to be discarded as medical waste and this happens in about 99% of births. This is rather a shocking statistic in that cord blood stem cells have been shown to be a good source of 'blood forming' stem cell for transplant, especially in children, but they are still being discarded globally, and on an industrial scale, due to either ignorance or complacency or both.

Public or Private Cord Blood Storage?

There is no easy answer to this conundrum. Not everyone can afford private cord blood storage, and many people are either totally unaware of the technology or are aware of it but mistrust it because of the many stories and scandals which have been reported in the past in stem cell technology. The stem cell industry has been its' own worst enemy in the past and that reputation sticks. Private cord blood storage is therefore either out of reach or unattractive for many people because of financial or technical concerns and misconceptions.

Private cord blood banks often attend baby shows where parents to be can see everything they might ever need for their baby. When speaking to parents to be at such shows, it is clear that a highly expensive baby buggy or the latest baby gizmo is a much more attractive proposition than the rather nebulous collection and storage of cord blood. I understand this psychology of the parents to be and most private cord blood banks, despite spending millions on marketing, fail to convince parents to be that private cord blood is a useful option for their family.

Public healthcare providers (for example the NHS) do not have the funds to set up widescale public cord blood collection and storage. This is because public cord blood collection, processing and storage are not properly understood or valued by politicians and decision makers in any country worldwide. There is a considerable amount of work needed before the public cord blood service in any Country becomes an effective life-saving process.

Discarding the cord blood at the birth of a baby is a cheap and easy option although the incineration bill sent to most hospitals for the destruction of medical waste is enormous and arguably bad for the environment (most medical waste is burnt in an incinerator). Cord blood is a valuable medical resource and it should not be incinerated.

Cord Blood Guidance

This is, as you can see, is a confusing subject but the purpose of this book is to inform and to provide guidance where needed, so here goes with some guidance:

If a young couple wish to store their cord blood privately for family use, and they have the money to do so, then these are some points to consider:

- Ideally it is not just a matter of money but in reality the cost of private cord blood storage is very high in all Countries and new parents, as mentioned above, often prefer to spend such amounts on the latest fashionable baby buggy or another baby 'essentials' which are far more visible than the slightly ethereal private cord blood storage which cannot be seen or held by anyone.
- Some people talk about private cord blood collection and storage as being 'biological insurance' or 'health insurance'. This terminology was created by journalists and marketing people and I was unfortunately 'quoted' as saying this in an article in the Telegraph in 2004. I have never agreed with or supported this terminology. Private cord blood storage is neither of these. It is a scientific process by which families can pay to have stem cells collected and stored for use in their family if needed. Wrapping it in unnecessary jargon and clever marketing speak only confuses the matter.
- There is a slight trend, which is very welcome, in some families for grandparents to pay for private cord blood storage (assuming that they are lucky enough to have disposable income) as a gift to the new baby. This is an interesting trend as grandparents have in the past received cord blood stem cell transplants from cord blood stored privately for the family!
- The ethereal privately stored cord blood, which no one can see or hold, becomes extremely important and visible when a family member needs it for transplant. I have been involved in several cord blood transplants over the years using privately stored cord blood and all of these families would agree that it was money well spent. These transplants have mostly been to parents, siblings, grandparents and even aunts and uncles. The success rate for these transplants is about 70% as it is for bone marrow stem cell transplants. When the transplant fails it us usually as a result of bleeding or infection or complications arising from conditioning or anti-rejection medication.

The other side of the coin of course is that privately stored cord blood is most likely to stay stored and not be needed by anyone in the family. This is the basis of the main argument which many people put forward against private cord blood storage. The simple answer to this objection is that if people choose to utilise private cord blood storage then they do so after providing informed consent for the process. This informed consent includes a clear understanding of the fact that the privately stored cord blood may never be needed for family use. There is also the matter of the developing applications for cord blood in the future, such as the treatment of cerebral palsy which *could* make private cord blood storage even more important. Nevertheless, cord blood for these applications could arguably be obtained from public banks (assuming that the public banks have the capacity to provide such cord blood units) which at present they do not.

Despite all of this, if an informed decision is made to go ahead with private cord blood collection and storage then the next problem is which company to choose?

There are hundreds, possibly thousands, of private cord blood banks worldwide. There is even a website (parentsguidecordblood.org) which lists all cord blood banks (public and private) around the world and provides useful and reliable information to people considering private cord blood storage. All of the private cord blood banks have shiny, impressive websites and all of them claim to be 'the best' and to have the 'most experience' and 'best technology'. You may sense my lack of appreciation of these claims; they are in general terms nonsense and are best ignored.

This confusion seems to mount but the following suggestions will help anyone interested in private cord blood storage to decide which company to use:

This next piece of advice may sound obvious, but it is very important:

• Select a private cord blood bank which is close to your delivery hospital so that the cord blood can be available for processing and storage within 24 hours of collection (at the birth of the baby). There are several private cord blood banks in the UK so this should be fairly easy to achieve. In actual fact many private cord blood banks in the UK get most of their business from Europe, the Middle East and even the Far East and report good quality cord blood on arrival in the UK. In order to achieve this, most UK private cord blood banks set a maximum transit time of 72 hours on cord blood collection from the delivery of the baby to arrival in the processing and storage laboratory. This extended transit time has been validated (shown to be safe) by the private cord blood banks but the key thought here is that the shorter the transit time, the better for your cord blood and setting your own maximum of 24 hours transit time should give plenty of leeway for delays along the way. Private cord blood banks will however, push the idea of a 72 hour maximum delivery period very strongly in order to maximise the amount and scope of their international business. Despite this, pushing the transit time to the limit is potentially bad for the stem cells in the cord blood and should ideally be avoided. It is interesting to note that most public cord blood banks set a maximum transit time of 12-24 hours. I wonder why that may be? Might it be that shorter transit times are better for the stem cells? I think it could be.

If the transit time goes to 73 hours, for example many private cord blood banks will still argue that processing and storage is still possible as they do not want to lose the processing and storage fees. This is bad practice. If a validated limit has been set, and something falls outside of that limit, then the cord blood collection should be rejected. However, this does not happen because most private cord blood banks are only interested in profit and will happily store inadequate or clinically useless cord blood on the basis that 'it might be useful in future advances in stem cell technology'. This is nonsense, do not accept this argument. The same applies to other limits set in science and to ignore these limits is very poor practice and could even be dangerous is some circumstances such as the cord blood unit being unsuitable when urgently needed and thawed for transplant.

- When you have selected a possible private cord blood bank, which is a sensible distance from your delivery hospital, then ask them when they started their business, how many cord blood units they have stored and how many cord blood units they have released for transplant?

The answers to these questions need to be that the company has a good well established history (ideally greater than 10 years old), it should have the experience of at least 1000 customers who have already stored their cord blood with them and they should have transplanted at least 0.1% (1 in a 1000) of the total number of cord blood units they have stored. One note of caution here is that many private cord blood banks exaggerate the number of cord blood units they have stored and it is virtually impossible to get reliable data from the private cord blood sector. Public cord blood banks tend to report the number of cord blood units they have stored more reliably.

If the private cord blood bank you are considering cannot either get close to or exceed these numbers, then they are probably inexperienced and *you do not want to be part of their learning curve*. The problem with this of course, is that the companies know these key quality indicators very well and may simply lie to get your business. If you become concerned then ask to visit the cord blood bank to see the facility and ask for information on which hospitals the transplants took place. You could also ask friends if they have privately stored cord blood and if so with which company? If you cannot obtain the information you need on a given private cord blood bank then look elsewhere. A private cord blood bank which avoids questions or provides vague, un-substantiated answers should be dismissed as unsuitable.

Whole or Processed?

This may sound a little strange, but it is possible to store cord blood without any processing (*i.e.* the total volume of cord blood collected, without any processing apart from the addition of the cryoprotectant, is frozen and stored). It is also possible to process the cord blood into a 25mL volume containing concentrated stem cells and then to freeze. Fig. (**6**) shows a 25mL volume cord blood stem cell unit. It is interesting to note that the first ever cord blood transplant used whole blood (*i.e.* no processing). The gold standard today however is the 25mL processed method largely because transplant centres prefer this form and the smaller volumes are more easily and effectively stored in cord blood banks. Nevertheless, it should also be noted that most transplant centres will also accept frozen whole cord blood if there is no other option. Some private cord blood banks offer both options and on balance, based on the current evidence and usage, it is worth going for the 25mL processed method if possible.

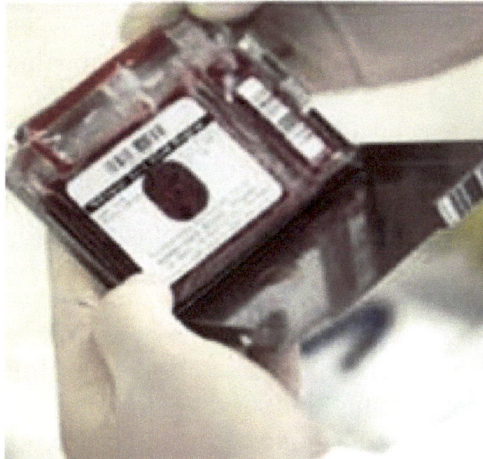

Fig. (6). Most cord blood stem cells are stored in 25mL bags.

More Questions

Assuming your chosen private cord blood bank passes these first questions the next step is to ask what accreditation and licensing they have?

• The important thing to understand here is that no cord blood bank should be operating unless they have their country specific licensing and/or accreditation and it is in fact illegal to do so in many countries. In the UK, for example, all cord blood banks (public and private) must be licensed to operate by the Human Tissue Authority (HTA) for a process called Human Application. Please note that a Research License from the HTA *does not* give the company the right to collect, process and store cells for human use. It is, as the name suggests, a license which allows a company to carry out research on human cells. The bottom line on this is that the private cord blood bank must have the appropriate license to practice in any given country. If they do not then they must be avoided at all costs, and reported to the authorities if they are attempting to enrol clients without a license.

- The second aspect here is accreditation, which is not compulsory, but it shows that the private cord blood bank has taken the time and effort to obtain further review of their systems and to obtain additional approval of their policies, procedures and organisation. There are many types of accreditation globally such as the International Organisation for Standardisation (ISO), the Joint Accreditation Committee ISCT Europe and EBMT (JACIE), the American Association of Blood Banks (AABB) and the Foundation for the Accreditation of Cellular Therapy (FACT). All of these accreditation bodies focus on what is known as Quality Management in the company. An effective Quality Management System *must* be used in the cord blood bank to ensure the quality and safety of the stored cord blood. Accreditation by any or all of these is a further indication of the commitment and professionalism of the private cord blood bank.
- It is also important to consider the qualifications and background of the scientific staff at the private cord blood clinic. The lead scientist should have at least 10 years' experience in cell therapy and ideally have a post-graduate degree in stem cell technology. There should also be a medically qualified advisor to the cord blood bank.

Once all of these questions have been answered, and boxes have been ticked to your satisfaction, it is important to understand that enrolling yourself for private cord blood collection, processing and storage and paying the deposit (which is usually non-refundable) does not guarantee the cord blood collection will take place. One reason for this is that your delivery hospital (especially in the UK) may not allow private cord blood collection on their premises. This is something you should confirm with your delivery hospital *before* paying any deposit to the private cord blood bank. In the UK and many other countries cord blood is collected on behalf of private cord blood banks by trained and competent external phlebotomists who are *not* hospital staff. This usually involves the placenta and cord being handed to the phlebotomist after the placenta has been delivered and the phlebotomist takes the placenta and cord to a separate room to collect the cord blood and cord tissue if needed. The fee for this service is payable by the cord blood clients and is usually part of the overall cost of collection, processing and storage. Please note that in the UK and in many other countries the husband or birthing partner of the pregnant women is **not** allowed to collect the cord blood even if they are medically qualified.

Another reason that cord blood collection may not be possible is because of medical problems during or after the delivery of the baby. The safety of the mother and baby is paramount and this may result in no cord blood being collected. This is a decision which will be made by the medical team caring for the mother and baby. Even if the cord blood is collected then the volume of cord blood obtained may be too low (usually anything less than 100mL is considered too low by most cord blood banks) to be useful in any future transplantation. If this happens then the cord blood bank will advise you accordingly and many of them may refund processing and storage fees (check the agreement with the private cord blood bank which you signed which will detail when a refund is possible). Be very wary of any cord blood banks which advise you to store cord blood which has a low volume (less than 100 mL) and a low cell count (less than 3 hundred million total nucleated cells) on arrival at the private cord blood bank. The rationale often put forward by private cord blood banks is that 'in the future low volume and low cell count cord blood collections may be useful'. *This is wishful thinking, marketing speak and nonsense.* Such cord blood collections have no future clinical value and if you are advised to continue with processing and storage despite low volume and low cell count this is simply the private cord blood bank optimising their income by storing a clinically useless cord blood units. Low volume and low cell count cord blood collections are automatically rejected by public cord blood banks and it is also worth noting that the definition and limits of low volume and low cell count in public cord blood banks are much higher than the same parameters in private cord blood banks. This means that there are very many cord blood units stored in private cord blood banks which are either borderline or useless in terms of clinical utility but nevertheless the owners of these poor, clinically useless cord blood units have still paid processing and storage fees and will continue to pay annual storage fees. Please beware!

You should also be aware that the mother has to have blood taken at the time of delivery of the baby to screen for infectious diseases such as HIV and Hepatitis. This is usually taken either by the hospital staff or by the phlebotomist who collected your cord blood. If the mother is unhappy, unwilling or unable to have this blood taken after the baby is delivered then please do not sign up for cord blood collection as cord blood cannot be processed and stored without these tests being carried out and coming back negative. The maternal blood, in the UK, can be collected for a period of up to 7 days following the birth if the cord blood was collected but maternal blood was unavailable at the time. This may not apply in other Countries.

To Clamp or Not to Clamp? That is the Question…

Another interesting, and perhaps slightly unusual, debate which has arisen recently on the subject of cord blood collection is that of umbilical cord clamping. This refers to the clamp which is placed on the umbilical cord after the baby is born in readiness for the umbilical cord to be cut. Every parent will be very familiar with this process.

Some people claim that the timing of this clamping is important as if the cord is clamped too quickly after the birth of the baby then this may prevent the baby from receiving all of the umbilical cord blood it needs. The scientific evidence for this is at best contradictory but it is powerful argument that the baby may be deprived of blood it needs by rapid cord clamping. Some people even advocate that the umbilical cord should not be clamped for several minutes after the birth of the baby when the circulation between the baby and the placenta has stopped. The fact is that cord clamping is irrelevant in relation to cord blood collection. Cord blood can be collected whenever the client and healthcare professionals allow it to be collected and there does not need to be an argument about this. There does, of course, need to be some cord blood there to collect as if it is left more than 5 minutes after delivery of the placenta then the blood in the placenta will all be clotted and the cord blood collection is likely to fail or result in a low volume/low cell count collection which should be rejected by the cord blood bank. Stem cell banks should not interfere with or dictate clamping times. This is a matter for the mother, her partner and the healthcare workers caring for her.

The UK Royal Colleges

A final thought on the public/private cord blood debate is to consider the opinions on cord blood collection in the UK which come from the Royal College of Obstetricians and Gynaecologists (RCOG) and the Royal College of Midwives (RCM). Other Countries have similar opinions from medical professional bodies. The UK organisations (RCOG and RCM) advise their members (obstetricians and midwives) on their clinical practice and both currently advise that private cord blood collection should not be encouraged. Their reason is that they believe that private cord blood is unlikely to be used and if stem cells are needed in the family then this can be sourced from public banks. As a result, the private cord blood storage industry in the UK is very weak (less than 1% of UK deliveries) and it actually relies on business from overseas to stay operational. In North America, where all patients receive unbiased information about private cord blood banking during their pregnancy, cord blood for private storage is collected in about 3% of deliveries. Donation of cord blood to the public banks is also better in North America because of better funding and infrastructure.

In summary private cord blood collection, processing and storage is a good idea assuming that the cost can be covered by the family and that the people using the service fully understand the benefits and limitations of the process. There are no guarantees that privately stored cord blood will either be needed or useful in the family in question but if it is needed in the family then it could be extremely useful, even life-saving.

Donation of cord blood to a public bank for use by anyone in need is a fantastic, altruistic act and it is more likely to be used to save a life globally. The donor infrastructure is however relatively weak in most Countries and further future investment is needed to optimise the public cord blood service. The availability of donated cord blood stem cells on an international basis will save lives and ultimately save money as patients in need recover and go back to their role in society. Politicians take note!

Discarding cord blood as medical waste is a global scandal resulting in the loss of valuable, life-saving stem cells on a daily basis. Education and funding should be put into place to reduce these daily losses to the population of the world. This is a matter for politicians on a global basis to discuss and to develop a coherent strategy but they will not do so until this subject is brought into the public consciousness, the media also needs to help and patient pressure to store and not discard cord blood is needed.

Umbilical Cord Blood Plasma

There is another component of cord blood, which is discarded even when cord blood stem cells are collected, and this is the plasma in cord blood. Plasma is the straw-coloured liquid which can be seen when any blood sample is centrifuged. In 2018 a research group in America showed that the plasma (no cells involved here) from umbilical cord blood could potentially help in the treatment of neurodegenerative disease. This effect is attributed to the many growth factors and other chemicals which are present in umbilical cord blood plasma which have the potential to interact with the central nervous system. Further workers in 2019 showed that umbilical cord blood plasma can have considerable benefits in the treatment of an animal model Parkinson's disease.

Umbilical cord blood plasma and its' future use in clinical practice is far from clear but more research is needed. We may be discarding a product which can help the ever increasing number of people suffering from the various types of neurodegenerative disease in our society.

KEY POINTS OF CHAPTER 4

- There are private cord blood banks collecting and storing cord blood for family use only, a fee is paid for the service.
- There are public cord blood banks collecting and storing cord blood for use by anyone in need, no fee is paid to the donor for this service.
- The chance of using a privately stored cord blood unit for a family member is low.
- Most of the cord blood available at birth is discarded as medical waste on a global scale.
- Great care is needed when choosing a private cord blood bank to ensure the safety and clinical efficacy of the stored cord blood.
- Cord blood plasma could be useful in the future treatment of neurodegenerative disease.

CHAPTER 5

That's a Nice Vein

(The introduction and use of peripheral blood stem cells)

Blood is a very special juice.
Johann Wolfgang von Goethe

Summary: This chapter considers the impact which has been made by the introduction of peripheral blood stem cell transplantation into routine clinical practice for the treatment of leukaemia and other blood disorders. The process helps in the collection of 'blood-forming' stem cells from bone marrow, and peripheral blood stem cell transplantation has now become the first-line treatment for most blood disorders.

PERIPHERAL BLOOD STEM CELLS

The introduction of the use of peripheral blood (taken from blood in the veins) stem cells in 1986 into routine clinical practice for the treatment of leukaemia and blood disorders represented a quantum change in the practice of bone marrow stem cell transplantation. The basic principle here is that adult 'blood-forming' stem cells normally live in our bone marrow (mostly in the pelvis and the long bones such as those in the thigh and lower leg). In order to harvest these stem cells for transplantation, it is necessary to carry out multiple puncture sites under general anaesthetic, from the pelvis. This is a relatively painful process which also carries the normal risks associated with a general anaesthetic, along with potential problems from bleeding or infection. Nevertheless, the traditional bone marrow harvest was critical in the early development of 'blood-forming' stem cell transplantation, and this process has saved thousands of lives globally.

The technology used in peripheral blood stem cell harvesting is very different from that used in a 'traditional' bone marrow harvest. The target cells for the collection are still the same 'blood-forming' stem cells which normally sit in the bone marrow, but peripheral blood stem cell technology enables a much easier collection of these stem cells making the whole process less traumatic for the donor, less risky for the donor and more cost-effective both for the donor, recipient and healthcare provider.

The key behind this technology is the ability to make 'blood-forming' stem cells leave the bone marrow and enter the peripheral circulation. This has been achieved by using a combination of medications which reduce the 'stickiness' of 'blood-forming' stem cells and allow them to enter the general circulation from the bone marrow. Once in the general circulation, these 'blood-forming' stem cells can be collected using a process called apheresis. In straight forward terms, apheresis is a very specialised centrifuge that can separate the stem cells from the rest of the blood cells. The process of apheresis is carried out by specially trained nurses or technicians as a 'day case' in hospital.

Following 'blood-forming' stem cell mobilisation into the peripheral blood by the use of medication, the patient is attached to an apheresis machine which draws blood from the patient and the patients' blood, containing stem cells, flows into the apheresis machine. The apheresis machine then separates the stem cells from the rest of the blood cells in the patients' blood. It keeps back the stem cells in a collection bag in the apheresis machine and returns all of the other blood cells and plasma back to the patient.

The stem cells obtained from the apheresis machine can then be frozen for later use either for the patient themselves or can be donated to another person. When the stem cells are later used by the patients themselves, this is referred to as an 'auto-transplant' or 'autologous transplant'. The scenario of an autologous transplant is usually when the patient has a blood disease that needs a stem cell transplant. When the stem cells collected by the apheresis machine, the patient receives treatment for the disease (*e.g.*, chemotherapy and/or radiotherapy), and once the treatment is complete and the disease has been eradicated, the patient receives their own stem cells back in a transplant as described earlier.

When the stem cells are donated to another person, this is referred to as an 'allo-transplant' or an 'allogeneic transplant'. Allogeneic transplantation from an unrelated donor to a recipient patient still requires the tissue match between donor and recipient in the same way as the bone marrow stem cells. This is because peripheral blood stem cells are just bone marrow stem cells which have been mobilised into the peripheral circulation and have exactly the same biology as they do when they are collected from bone marrow directly.

This collection of peripheral blood stem cells from unrelated donors has resulted in a revolution in stem cell donation because of the relative ease in which a donor (or indeed the transplant patient themselves in the case of an autologous transplant) can make their donation. Previously, a donor would have to undergo a bone marrow harvest under general anaesthesia, but now they can donate their stem cells by a relatively easy and non-invasive process, which makes stem cell donation more attractive to altruistic donors.

Organisations such as Anthony Nolan in the UK now collect stem cells from their donors using apheresis, and they even carry out the initial tissue typing by a simple 'cheek swab', making the process quick and easy. The potential donor is sent to a specially designed swab, which is used by the donor to collect a few cheek cells from inside the side of the mouth. The DNA in these cells is then examined in the laboratory, and from this, the basic tissue type of the donor can be assessed, and this is sufficient to match the donor to a potential recipient. If the transplant is to proceed further, blood tests from the donor are needed, but the initial 'cheek swab' is a great way to get potential donors onto the database and has made the initial donor registration process much more attractive to prospective donors. This means that more potential donors are now on the database, which in turn means that more lives can be saved.

Potential Problems

As with all things in life, nothing is perfect (not even me), and the peripheral blood stem cell process is no exception. The main problem which can arise is that the medication fails to release enough stem cells from the bone marrow, or it might even fail to release any stem cells at all. This can be a particular problem when older patients (40 years plus) try to undergo peripheral blood stem cell mobilisation. In general terms, the older the patient, the less likely successful stem cell mobilisation can be achieved. This means that not enough stem cells are collected for treatment, which of course, can have a big impact on the patient, especially if it is an auto-transplantation (using the patient's own bone marrow) with no back-up source of stem cells. The apheresis technology is also relatively expensive, and the people who operate it need specialised training, and finally, children do not tolerate apheresis very well. In general terms, apheresis is not used when a child needs a stem cell transplant using his or her own cells. It is, of course, possible for an adult to donate peripheral blood stem cells for the treatment of a child.

Despite these potential problems, peripheral blood stem cells are by far the most common treatment route for leukaemia and blood disorders and are considered by most practitioners as the 'gold standard'. This means that you can feel safe and re-assured if you are a patient undergoing peripheral blood stem cell transplantation in a recognised treatment centre.

Improved Mobilisation Technology

The mobilisation of peripheral blood stem cells has been improved recently, especially in those patients where mobilisation is difficult, by the use of a medication called a 'CXCR4 antagonist'. This compound (which has the trade name Plerixafor) interferes with the attachment of stem cells in the bone marrow, which in turn makes them easier to mobilise for apheresis. This medication has been shown to be very useful in patients suffering from lymphoma and myeloma, who often find it very difficult to mobilise stem cells from the bone marrow, which previously has resulted in failed treatments for some patients. The CXCR4 antagonists will no doubt play an increasing role in routine stem cell mobilisation in the future.

Clinical Trials Using Peripheral Blood Stem Cells

At the time of writing, there were 109 clinical trials recruiting volunteers and most of these are assessing potential improvements to peripheral blood stem cell technology especially refining a procedure known as haploidentical transplantation. When a patient receives a haploidentical transplant, the donor cells are usually obtained from a close family member; ideally, parents or siblings, and the match between the donor and recipient patient is usually around 50%. The potential rejection problems which would occur following haploidentical transplantation are then controlled by giving extra chemotherapy after the transplant and infusions of white cells to regulate the immune response after the transplant. By giving this additional treatment, the method of haploidentical transplantation has become very common. This development is largely due to a better understanding of the process of transplantation, the development of improved chemotherapy medication and the development of 'cell removal' technology, which selectively removes the cells involved in rejection from the donor peripheral blood stem cells. The fact that a close family member will almost always be a suitable haploidentical donor makes the future development and general application of this technology extremely important. In some transplant centres, haploidentical transplantation using peripheral blood stem cells is the first line of treatment, and the outcomes are very good.

In summary, 'blood-forming' peripheral blood stem cells are used around the World to treat blood disorders and are considered to be the 'gold standard'. Their use requires highly skilled healthcare workers and state of the art equipment and facilities to ensure a good outcome. The application of 'blood-forming' peripheral blood stem cells to haploidentical transplantation is very important and will be increasingly used as a first-line treatment for blood disorders.

KEY POINTS OF CHAPTER 5

- Peripheral blood stem cells are now the 'gold standard' for blood-forming stem cell transplantation.
- The collection process is less invasive than a bone marrow harvest.
- Many donors now undergo peripheral blood stem cell harvesting instead of bone marrow harvesting making the process more attractive to altruistic donors.
- Peripheral blood stem cell technology requires highly trained healthcare workers and state of the art equipment.
- Haploidentical transplantation (using 'blood-forming' peripheral blood stem cells from a close relative) is now widely practiced with great success.
- Peripheral blood mobilization technology is advancing rapidly to improve the number of stem cells collected.

CHAPTER 6

The Vatican and More

(Concepts and controversies surrounding human embryonic stem cells)

And many false prophets shall rise, and shall deceive many.
Peter J. Tanous

Summary: This chapter examines the debates, and sometimes the hope *versus* hype, which surrounds embryonic stem cells and their potential use in clinical transplantation. The use of human embryos in stem cell technology creates many strong opinions from a surprisingly wide range of people. This chapter explores the pros and cons of embryonic stem cells and gives an overview of the possible future for embryonic stem cells.

A COMPLEX DEBATE

It is sometimes very surprising who becomes involved in debates about stem cell transplantation and regenerative medicine. The most likely people to be interested are scientists, clinicians, the media, regulatory authorities, and, of course, the many companies who produce the equipment and chemicals needed for the stem cell manipulation and transplantation process.

Occasionally, potential patients, actual patients or celebrities have become involved in the debate. For example, Christopher Reeve (of Superman fame) became a great advocate for embryonic stem cell technology following his tragic spinal injury. Unfortunately, human embryonic stem cells are yet to be used to treat spinal damage, and they were never made available (at least they were never reported as being made available) to Christopher before his unfortunate death.

There are also private clinics worldwide that provide stem cell therapy and who are very vociferous, if not often misinformed, misled, or simply led by profit, about their chosen type of stem cells. Such companies have a clear financial interest to promote the use of stem cell technology, which may persuade them that providing proof of safety and efficacy of their stem cell products is a hindrance to their progress.

The clinicians, scientists and others working in stem cell technology usually get together in international conferences (which in the post-Covid19 future will hopefully happen virtually) to discuss new ideas and confirm old ideas. These are often the most constructive discussions which focus on stem cell facts and not hype and myth. The development of embryonic stem cells, derived from human embryos as a potential source of stem cells for clinical use, has brought many more people into the debate, including religious leaders of all faiths, medical ethicists, medical lawyers and of course, the media and journalists also want to join the party!

Human Embryonic Stem Cell Production

In order to properly understand why there is so much interest from so many different people about human embryonic stem cells, it is necessary to understand the basics of their creation and the potential of their use.

Embryonic stem cells are extracted from a human embryo five days following fertilisation of the human egg with human sperm. This fertilisation process must be carried out in a laboratory and is, therefore, always part of an *in vitro* fertilisation (IVF) procedure. The embryo at this five-day stage after fertilisation is called a blastocyst, and it is a hollow ball of cells (consisting of about 120 cells in total), and it is about 0.1mm in diameter. Such an embryo can just be seen by the naked eye, but under a low power microscope, the beauty of the blastocyst can be clearly seen. The walls of the ball which forms a blastocyst are uniform apart from one area where the cells are thicker, this is called the inner cell mass. The inner cell mass is the area of the embryo, which will eventually develop into the baby, and the thinner, more uniform area (the trophoblast) of the blastocyst will develop into the placenta and membranes of the pregnancy, such as the amniotic membrane. In order to obtain human embryonic stem cells, it is necessary to dissect the inner cell mass from the rest of the human embryo and grow the dissected cells in the laboratory for several more days. It is this process, which results in the destruction of a human embryo and the creation of human embryonic stem cells, which has sparked the medical, financial, legal and religious interest of so many people and created worries in others.

The Human Embryo

The key thing to remember here is that a human embryo is a small collection of cells that is the basis of human life. Some theologians (most notably past and possibly present Popes) and ethicists object to the deliberate destruction of human embryos even when the purpose of the destruction is to obtain human embryonic stem cells to treat other human beings in need. They see it as the death of human life (even killing or murder in some minds) to treat another human life; it is viewed as unacceptable to them.

It is also very important to ask where the human embryos are obtained for the creation of human embryonic stem cells. The answer is that all embryos come from 'unwanted' frozen human embryos in IVF clinics around the world. These are most usually from successful IVF treatment cycles where the parents have achieved the family they desire, and the frozen embryos remaining at the IVF clinic are no longer needed for fertility treatment. The parents have the option in most countries to either simply destroy the frozen embryos, donate them to another couple or donate them to research where the primary purpose will be to create human embryonic stem cells. This situation is unique in embryonic stem cell technology, where the 'donor' is a human embryo, and the embryo cannot give informed consent for the process. Informed consent is obtained from the parents of the embryos prior to any manipulations to create embryonic stem cells. This represents the best option available to ensure consent in the embryonic stem cell process.

All of the other stem cell donors discussed in this book are either from adult human donors who have given informed consent themselves, or the stem cells are obtained from the 'waste products' of childbirth, from fat liposuction or from teeth, which would otherwise be discarded. The consent process in all of these is very clear, and in these cases, the patients from which the 'waste products' are obtained have given their informed consent to further use their tissue.

It is clearly impossible for a frozen human embryo to give its' consent for anything, and for many people, who view the human embryo as an individual human, this is a serious cause for concern. Some people even consider the dissection and destruction of a human embryo to obtain human embryonic stem cells as a form of 'murder' in that the potential for human life has been taken away. This is a complex debate that is far from concluded even today and perhaps will never be resolved to the satisfaction of everyone involved.

The stem cells obtained from a human embryo are different from other types of stem cells in that they have the potential to form any type of tissue in the body and could therefore be used, in theory, to treat an almost never-ending list of diseases. This fires up the imagination, especially that of the media, that embryonic stem cells could be the panacea for disease. Sadly, this is not true, and it is not even close to being true for the reasons which are discussed below.

Is There an Elephant in The Room?

The large and overpowering 'elephant in the room' when talking about human embryonic stem cells is that to obtain these stem cells requires the destruction of a human embryo, and are there enough human embryos available for this purpose? The answer to this question is no. This means that putting ethical, legal and religious objections to one side; if we had clear, tested and safe applications for embryonic stem cells for lots of different diseases, then there would simply not be enough human embryos in fertility clinics (around the World) to provide the embryonic stem cells needed for treatment. Some people suggest that human embryos could be created specifically to extract embryonic stem cells. This is the thin end of a very nasty legal, ethical, moral and religious wedge, which we must avoid at all costs.

The Vatican has also pitched in to the debate with the opinion that embryonic stem cell technology is unacceptable in their eyes and instead, they strongly support the future use of adult and fetal stem cells, especially cord blood, such as those described in this book. This opinion is clearly driven largely by religious belief relating to the sanctity of human life. In actual fact, this Vatican opinion also agrees with most stem cell researchers and practitioners who believe that adult and fetal stem cells are the future in the Regeneration Promise and that embryonic stem cells will only play a limited role, if any role at all.

Clinical Trials

At the time of writing, there were 10 clinical trials enrolling patients into projects related mainly to the treatment of disease in the eye. It seems that human embryonic stem cells are good at repairing a structure called the retina in the eye, which is the light-sensitive tissue which forms the basis of vision. The clinical trials are ongoing, but if they prove that human embryonic stem cells are safe and effective in the treatment of eye disease, then this could possibly be a 'niche' application for these cells. Only time will tell, but even if this 'niche' application becomes routine clinical practice, there still remains the availability problem and overall acceptability of using these cells, which will need to be solved to the satisfaction of everyone.

A FINAL NOTE OF OPTIMISM!

In May 2020, it was reported by a group in Japan that liver cells, derived from human embryonic stem cells, had been used to treat a newborn baby who was suffering from severe life-threatening liver disease. The concept here was to use the liver cells derived from human embryonic stem cells as a 'bridging treatment'. The baby had to have a liver transplant to achieve a full cure, but the liver cells derived from human embryonic stem cells provided support for the baby until a transplant could be carried out. Babies otherwise often die from the toxic effects of their malfunctioning liver, so this treatment could be a future lifesaver. Whilst this is great work, the objections to, and availability of, human embryonic stem cells still remain.

KEY POINTS OF CHAPTER 6

- Embryonic stem cells could, in theory, be used to treat a wide range of diseases.
- Embryonic stem cells are created by the destruction of a human embryo, which raises many objections to their routine use.
- Clinical trials are underway to assess the possibility of using human embryonic stem cells to make light-sensitive cells in the eye.
- Liver cells derived from human embryonic stem cells may be useful in the treatment of liver disease.

CHAPTER 7

No One Likes the Dentist

(Ideas behind dental pulp stem cells)

I always wanted to be a dentist from the time I was in high school, and I was accepted to dental school in the spring of 1972. I was planning to go, but after the Olympics, there were other opportunities.
Mark Spitz

Summary: This chapter summarises the amazing progress which has been made from the discovery that there are 'tissue forming' stem cells inside teeth which can be 'extracted' and potentially used as the basis of future therapies. The process of dental stem cell collection and storage is described along with an overview of the potential applications of dental pulp stem cells.

OFF TO SEE THE DENTIST

A trip to see the dentist can mean many things. Fear, apprehension, relief (if you have toothache) and sometimes elation when the diagnosis of 'all clear' is given for another six months. Whatever your emotions, there is a relatively new concept in dentistry which has caught the imagination of stem cell scientists and increasingly some dentists. This excitement comes from the discovery of the presence of 'tissue forming' stem cells *inside* teeth which can be collected, processed, stored and potentially used in the treatment of a range of diseases.

Milk and Adult Teeth

Everyone is familiar with 'milk teeth', which are the first teeth a child develops, and these 'milk teeth' naturally fall out around age 5-6 years and are then replaced by permanent 'adult teeth'. Researchers have shown that both 'milk teeth' and 'adult teeth' contain 'tissue forming' stem cells with the possible potential to be useful in regenerative medicine and even possibly in dentistry.

Milk Teeth Collection

When a child naturally loses a 'milk tooth', it is possible to collect the tooth, place it into a transport medium such as saline containing antibiotics, or even milk, and send it to a laboratory to be processed and frozen. On arrival at the laboratory, the tooth is split open to expose the internal tissue (called dental pulp) which contains the stem cells, and the whole opened tooth is then frozen using liquid nitrogen in a special freezing solution which protects the stem cells.

There are, however, some practical problems with the collection, processing and storage of 'milk teeth' which have possibly contributed to the general lack of uptake of such a service:

- Firstly, the tooth fairy is furious and is considering legal action.
- Secondly, a single 'milk tooth' contains very few stem cells, so as a practical proposition to provide stem cells in the numbers needed to be clinically useful, it would need several, if not all, of a child's 'milk teeth' to be collected and stored.
- Thirdly, most regulatory authorities require the donor of stem cells, in this case, a child, to undergo infectious disease screening at the time of donation. In practical terms, this means that the child would have to undergo a blood test and be screened for HIV, hepatitis and syphilis. This could be traumatic for some children and parents considering 'milk tooth' collections and storage.

In summary, 'milk teeth' stem cell collection and storage are not to be recommended at present because the cost and invasive testing of the child are not balanced by the benefits. 'Milk teeth' stem cells have no current clinical use, although they may be useful in future clinical trials, especially in the creation of bone in patients where the bone loss in the jaw is causing dental problems. It is likely that if such applications become routine, then the stem cells from many 'milk teeth' would either have to be pooled together to treat one patient or the stem cells would have to be expanded in the laboratory.

Stem Cells from Adult Teeth

The second area of interest in dental pulp stem cell technology involves those 'tissue forming' stem cells which have been shown to be present inside adult teeth. The proposal here is that when an adult has a *healthy* tooth extracted, either for impacted wisdom teeth or for orthodontic reasons (overcrowding), then the tooth can be sent for adult stem cell processing and storage following the same process described above for 'milk teeth'. The adult donor has to undergo infectious disease screening as described above but this is of course less invasive than doing this on a child and the blood could easily be taken at the time of extraction of the tooth. Adult teeth are of course physically larger than 'milk teeth', and as such, each adult tooth contains more stem cells and the potential of these stem cells to be useful in the future is slightly increased. There is still, however, considerable uncertainty as to whether or not adult teeth stem cells will have any useful application in the future. Therefore, there is no evidence to support collecting and storing adult teeth at present.

The relatively simple process of collecting and storing 'milk' and 'adult' teeth has resulted in the development of companies which specialise in tooth collection and storage, such as Bioeden in the UK. Tooth collection and storage have also now been added to the services provided by most private umbilical cord blood banks. This made the relatively low demand tooth collection and storage service a viable business proposition to existing cord blood banks as a service 'add on' and some companies even predicted significant profits from the service; these profits have yet to be materialised.

Are There Enough Stem Cells?

The main problem with both baby teeth and adult teeth in terms of stem cell therapy is that neither source contains very many stem cells. This means that to use these cells in current treatment or clinical trial procedures as 'tissue forming' stem cells would require either some sort of cell expansion in the laboratory prior to use or to pool the stem cells from many teeth. This would increase the number of stem cells available for treatment. The expansion would, however, be using chemicals and/or bioreactors to increase the cell numbers and this would make the final product a 'pharmaceutical'. This puts the expanded dental stem cell product into a category which requires a very high level of regulation.

Pooling the stem cells from several teeth is simple enough but this would rely on a person having several teeth stored which is unlikely. This is especially unlikely for 'adult' teeth unless both wisdom teeth have been stored or several teeth have been extracted for orthodontic reasons and stored. It is theoretically possible to collect all of the 'baby' teeth but in practice this is unlikely to happen. The parents of young children will understand why!

This makes the whole process unattractive as a source of 'tissue forming' stem cells for clinical use when tissue such as fat can provide the number of stem cells needed without any expansion.

Tooth Implants

The only scenario where teeth stem cells could *possibly* be used without expansion is surprisingly enough in dentistry. This is in the area of tooth implants which are becoming a very popular way to replace lost adult teeth. The concept here (without getting into too much gory dental surgery detail) is that the dentist screws an implant into the empty tooth socket and then attaches a permanent (artificial) replacement tooth to the implant. This sounds like a relatively easy procedure but a problem arises when the patient lost the tooth some time ago and now wants an implant. When a tooth is lost, the bone in the jaw which used to surround the tooth recedes to the point where there is not enough bone left into which the implant can be screwed. The current standard solution to this is to put 'artificial' bone (usually calcium phosphate based products and occasionally even donor bone from animals) into the socket where there has been bone loss and to wait for the natural production of new bone to take place. This might take several weeks or even months. In some patients new bone is not re-formed which means that the implant procedure cannot proceed. Assuming that adequate bone formation has been created by the artificial bone then the implant can be screwed into the new bone and the replacement tooth can be fitted.

It is possible that tooth stem cells (which are 'tissue forming' stem cells capable of making bone) could be used to promote bone formation for tooth implants which could result in better and quicker bone formation. The concept may be to mix the previously stored stem cells (or even donor tooth stem cells could be used) with the artificial bone and put this combination into the area where new bone formation is needed. As this is a very precise and local procedure, the number of stem cells from a tooth, without expansion, might be sufficient to promote quicker and better bone formation.

If this proves to be a safe and effective procedure then it may result in tooth stem cells being more relevant to routine dental practice. It is, of course, possible to use other types of 'tissue forming' stem cells from sources such as fat in this process, and at present, we do not know if these would be as good as tooth stem cells. More research is needed to understand these issues.

Clinical Trial

There is, at the time of writing, currently one clinical trial recruiting volunteers which is investigating the possible use of teeth stem cells to treat diabetes. This either reflects the lack of interest in teeth stem cells or an indication that the practical use of these cells is at best limited. I suspect the latter but I might be proven wrong.

KEY POINTS OF CHAPTER 7

- 'Milk teeth' and 'adult teeth' both contain stem cells which can be collected and stored for later use.
- The stem cells in teeth are 'tissue forming' and can make bone and connective tissue.

- At present, the clinical utility of these dental stem cells is extremely limited but in the future, they could become an important tool in regenerative medicine and dentistry especially in tooth implant technology.

CHAPTER 8

Who Are You Calling Fat?

(Ideas behind adipose or fat stem cells)

The devil has put a penalty on all things we enjoy in life. Either we suffer in health, or we suffer in soul, or we get fat.
Albert Einstein

Summary: This chapter describes the progress which has been made in the identification, collection, processing, storage and clinical use of fat or adipose stem cells. The technology is developing very rapidly and the application of adipose stem cells in both routine therapy and clinical trial is increasing rapidly.

FAT: GOOD OR BAD?

We all carry fat around and, in small amounts, it is essential for normal health. Many of our organs, especially the central nervous system, need fat in order to operate properly. Some nerves, for example, are covered in a 'fatty sheath', which provides insulation for the nerve impulse in the same way that plastic insulates an electrical cable. Loss or damage to this fatty covering in nerves results in serious diseases such as multiple sclerosis.

Nevertheless, due to poor diet, lack of exercise and an easy access to high fat food in some countries, many of the population are obese (carrying too much fat around) or morbidly obese (a patient who carries so much fat that there is a clear danger of serious life-threatening illness resulting from the excess fat). Fat therefore has a bad image and fat is generally seen as a bad thing with no real benefit. However, things might be changing.

The change has been driven by the discovery that fat contains 'tissue forming' stem cells which can be harvested and potentially used to treat a wide range of disease. Plastic surgeons have in fact been using the patients' own fat in reconstructive and cosmetic surgery for decades but the discovery of adipose (fat) stem cells opens up many new potential therapeutic options.

Liposuction

The initial studies on fat stem cells focussed on the fat which is collected when a person undergoes liposuction to remove excess fat from the abdomen. This is a surgical procedure, requiring a general anaesthetic, and it carries the usual risks of

bleeding and infection associated with such invasive procedures. Most liposuction procedures are carried out in private clinics as major public health care providers

such as the NHS tend to exclude the procedure (because it is considered to be a cosmetic procedure) unless it is required as a treatment of related diseases.

When a liposuction procedure is carried out, it is possible to obtain up to 5 litres of fat weighing up to 11 pounds. In the past, this fat has been discarded as medical waste but patients now have the option to send it on for processing and storage of the 'tissue forming' stem cells found in the fat. This storage is carried out by existing private cord blood banks who were quick to add fat to their range to produce another income stream.

Processing of Fat Stem Cells Using Enzymes

These amounts of fat, obtained from liposuction, do however present quite a challenge to the processing laboratories. Firstly, it requires expensive reagents and equipment to process the fat which make the overall process quite costly. Secondly, the processing involves the use of enzymes which are chemicals and which allow the release of the stem cells from the rest of the fat cells. The use of enzymes is not in itself a problem, in fact enzymes enable good collection of stem cells, but the regulatory authorities (such as the MHRA in the UK) view the use of chemicals such as enzymes as an increased level of manipulation. This increased manipulation using enzymes means that fat stem cells attract the attention of regulatory authorities who more usually regulate pharmaceuticals. This is not a problem in itself but the increased level of regulation, when using enzymes to process fat, results in increased costs in terms of regulatory, staffing, facilities and equipment costs. This increased cost makes the collection, processing and storage of fat stem cells using enzymes not really a practical proposition, and as such, has held back some developments in fat stem cell technology.

Processing of Fat Stem Cells Using A Mechanical Approach

A recent solution to this problem has been proposed by several researchers who have discovered that fat can be processed by mechanical means to extract the stem cells. This mechanical digestion of the fat commonly uses a selection of clinical grade blades (inside a sterile, small single use box) through which the fat is passed. This approach considerably simplifies the processing of fat and the extraction of fat stem cells. Mechanical processing of fat tissue takes away the extra regulation which enzyme treated fat stem cells attracted, which in turn reduces the cost of using fat stem cells.

This mechanical digestion technology is a major breakthrough in fat stem cell technology as it has changed the process from being complex and expensive to being relatively easy and cheap. Many physicians have, in fact, already used this mechanical digestion technology and have developed a system which can collect fat. Small amounts of fat (10-20mL) can be collected under local anaesthetic at the bedside or larger amounts in the operating theatre. The fat is then immediately processed using mechanical digestion technology and then immediately used either for cosmetic or regenerative applications (an autologous procedure). This simplification of fat stem cell therapy is extremely important because it brings the technology to a greater range of patients at a reduced cost with less processing intervention resulting in reduced regulatory requirements.

Caution is Needed

There is however a cautionary tale. There were 3 patients in Florida who were blinded after taking part in a 'clinical trial' using fat stem cells. These patients were enrolled into a 'clinical trial' run by the company involved and they were each asked to pay $5000 to take part in the trial. This request for payment should have rung a multitude of alarm bells because clinical trial volunteers should ***never be asked to pay to take part in the trial***. These unfortunate patients clearly did not know this and either ignored advice or made the mistake of not taking advice at this stage. *Always* take unbiased, independent advice if you are thinking of taking part in a clinical trial. These unfortunate people joined the 'clinical trial', paid their money, and received injections of their own 'processed' adipose stem cells into both eyes. The fact that they received treatments into both eyes at the same time is quite shocking. Even experienced ophthalmologists only treat one eye at a time to minimise unanticipated complications in both eyes and once again if the patients had taken advice then they would have had this fact highlighted. The outcome was that these three patients became permanently blind. This is a shocking example of malpractice in the stem cell industry. It also illustrates the extreme vulnerability of some patients who, in their desperation, can easily be drawn into a procedure which is dangerous and unproven.

Clinical Trials and 'Freeze Young'

Despite this horror story, adipose (fat) stem cells do have enormous potential when used properly either in tried and tested applications or in clinical trial. The 'tissue forming' stem cells found in adipose tissue could be particularly useful in the repair of bone, connective tissue (tendons and cartilage) and also in the regulation of the immune system which could be useful in diseases such as diabetes and multiple sclerosis. This makes fat stem cells very interesting in treating inflammatory diseases such as osteoarthritis.

At the time of writing, there have been 42 clinical trials using fat stem cells which have recruited patients and many of these focussed on the treatment of osteoarthritis. Most of these clinical trials have used autologous fat stem cells *i.e.* stem cells collected from the patient and used on that same patient. This avoids any possible rejection of the stem cells used in the treatment but in fact 'tissue forming' stem cells in general can be donated from person to person without a high risk of rejection. This is a biological property of all types of 'tissue forming' stem cells and it means that banks of 'tissue forming' stem cells could be used relatively easily in the future.

The advantage of this autologous approach to treatment is that we are all carrying around a good source of stem cells in our fat which can be collected and used for our own treatment when required. It is generally far better to use 'fresh' stem cells in this way rather than to rely on frozen stem cells which, because of the very fact that they have been frozen in liquid nitrogen and thawed for treatment, may not be as effective as fresh stem cells. The only downside of using your own stem cells when needed is that your stem cells age along with you. Patients who are older will have stem cells which are older and perhaps not as effective as younger stem cells. Some people suggest that younger people should store their stem cells when they are young for possible use later when they are older. This would mean that an older person could receive their own younger stem cells when needed and these stem cells might work better even when allowing for the fact that they have been frozen.

There is no strong evidence at present that this 'freeze young' proposal is effective, but from a basic science point of view, it seems to make sense. The critical point in this will be to ensure that the 'young' stem cells are frozen using the very best technology to minimise their long-term damage by freezing. Further research and clinical trials are needed to assess this important aspect of stem cell technology.

Fat Stem Cells and Osteoarthritis

The most popular diseases treated in these clinical trials include osteoarthritis and related joint disorders. This reflects the ability of fat stem cells to modulate the immune system (diseases such as arthritis can sometimes be caused by an over-active immune system causing inflammation) and also to repair cartilage in the diseased joint. Fat stem cells may also secrete chemicals which can promote natural repair in diseased joints.

Fat stem cells clearly have great potential in the Regeneration Promise, but at the same time, we have to proceed with caution to avoid potential harm. This is achieved by controlled clinical trials only and not by opportunistic 'snake-oil' salesmen promoting untested, unsafe technology to a vulnerable population.

KEY POINTS OF CHAPTER 8

- Fat has been shown to be a good source of 'tissue forming' stem cells.
- The processing method is important and ideally does not use enzymes so that the regulatory issues are minimised.
- Fat has been used in cosmetic surgery for many years and new stem cell therapies using fat stem cells are in clinical trials.
- As with all stem cell technology, caution is needed, as some people have already gone through major damage from poor treatment using fat stem cells.
- The freezing of fat stem cells of the patients when they are young, for use when they are older, may provide better results; however, this proposal has yet to be fully confirmed.

CHAPTER 9

A Human Touch

(The development and use of induced pluripotent stem cells)

Nothing eases suffering like a human touch.
Bobby Fischer

Summary: This chapter describes the development and potential applications of man-made stem cells called induced pluripotent stem cells (iPSC). The technology involved and the possibilities for research and therapy are described.

MAN-MADE

All of the stem cell achievements, advances, and disappointments so far described in this book have been made using human intuition, knowledge, determination, and sometimes good luck. The stem cells which have been described are all naturally occurring and their use has been a matter of discovery and clinical utilization. This has brought us to the point where we have considerable and increasing knowledge in stem cell technology, but there is clearly much more to be done.

This chapter considers a new type of stem cell, which is man-made. It is called an induced pluripotent stem cell (often called iPSC) and it is a 'tissue forming' stem cell capable, in theory, of producing all tissue types in the body similar to the properties of embryonic stem cells. This is why it has the term 'pluripotent' in its' name. This means that it can, in theory, make all of the tissues of the body. In order to create iPSC, researchers took the unusual step of making their starting point a natural skin cell. Skin cells can be obtained very easily either by a very quick and painless biopsy or even by a simple swab of the inside of the cheek. Even though there are stem cells in the skin itself (these skin stem cells regenerate the skin on a daily basis), it is not these stem cells which were of interest. The purpose is to obtain a normal cell which was easy to obtain and manipulate, making skin the obvious candidate. Many workers have since used blood cells as the starting point for iPSC, which is arguably easier than using skin. Once the scientists had the starting point of normal human skin or blood cell, the next challenge was to treat this cell to make it transform from a normal skin or blood cell to a 'tissue forming' stem cell. This transformation was achieved by using an 'inactivated' virus to introduce 4 new genes into the skin or blood cell. These 4 genes resulted in the cell changing from normal skin or blood to a 'tissue forming' stem cell.

This work caused great excitement in the stem cell community (so much excitement that the scientists involved were awarded a Nobel prize) because it meant that any patient needing 'tissue forming' stem cells for treatment could have them 'manufactured' on demand from their own normal tissue cells, in theory.

Good or Bad?

The production of iPSC, at first, sounded like the ultimate stem cell solution to the Regeneration Promise but it soon became clear that such manipulation of cells might not be quite as attractive. Two specific concerns were raised by many scientists; these are:

- The use of a virus to introduce new genes into skin or blood cells. People question whether the virus could place the 4 new genes in the correct place in the skin or blood cell and if the genes went into the wrong place, then would there be unforeseen problems? The answer, at present, to this question is that we do not really know but great caution is recommended. Any procedure which involves changing, replacing, or adding genes into a cell is potentially risky.
- The second criticism relates to the 4 genes themselves. Some of the genes used were genes known to be associated with malignant cancerous cells. The worry was that if these genes are introduced into normal cells, could they, at some point, form malignant cells? The answer, at present, is that the genes associated with malignant cancerous cells should be avoided where possible and many workers have developed alternative genes that enable iPSC development but are not associated with malignant disease. Once again, great caution is recommended.

Despite these concerns, research and development work has continued on iPSC with the development of different gene delivery systems and some workers even used different genes to create iPSC. These two changes began to make iPSC more readily accepted but the creation of iPSC is still controversial. This controversy becomes even stronger when the potential for clinical use of iPSC is discussed. For this reason, iPSCs have stayed in the research laboratory, rather than going immediately to a clinical trial, in order to properly assess their safety. If iPSCs eventually come into routine clinical use, then it will only be thorough clinical trials, to show evidence of safety and efficacy, which will ideally be carried out on a global multi-center scale.

Organoids

Despite the concerns surrounding the clinical use of iPSC, the use of these man-made stem cells in research has continued and is starting to show some very interesting possibilities.

One particular development in iPSC 'tissue forming' stem cell technology has been to use them as the basis for a technology called organoids. Organoids are created by first creating some iPSC as described above and then driving these iPSCs (using known chemicals and stimulatory molecules) to produce specific tissues, such as kidney, nerve or liver. The resultant tissue cells produced from iPSC start to cluster together to produce tiny versions of the organs they represent and this is known as an organoid. Organoids have several potential uses, such as the study of disease processes in organs, screening of pharmaceuticals, and even possibly, some role in therapy in the future, although there is still an enormous amount of work to be done before any therapeutic applications of iPSC organoids become a reality. It is possible, maybe even likely, that this may never happen.

Organoids which develop into testicular or ovarian tissue have been proposed as a potential source of gametes (sperm and eggs) to treat infertile patients. At present, this is just an interesting concept largely because of the extremely complicated biological and ethical issues raised by such a proposal. It could, for example, be possible to make testicular and ovarian organoids from the same person, obtain sperm and eggs and create an embryo and put this embryo back into the original cell donor (assuming that she was female). This kind of proposal raises so many concerns and objections that it is never likely to happen. This is a good thing.

It would even be theoretically possible to do this process to create iPSC derived sperm and eggs using a donor who has already gone through menopause or suffered an early menopause. Such ideas are wild, untested concepts at the moment, but if the technology develops, we may soon be faced with ethical dilemmas, about firstly, should research be allowed and secondly, should such technology be used in clinical practice? My thought at the moment is a clear 'no' to both of these questions, but only time will tell.

Clinical Trials

At the time of writing, there were 19 clinical trials recruiting volunteers using iPSC as the basis of the trial. These clinical trials cover a wide range of applications, from applications in the eye to neurological and heart disease. Some of these studies are trying to assess possible clinical applications, but most are trying to develop organoids, which will then be used as an experimental model of the disease.

KEY POINTS OF CHAPTER 9

- It is possible to make stem cells from normal skin or blood cells by introducing new genes into the skin cells.
- The initial genes used are associated with malignant cancers and alternative genes are needed to ensure safety.
- iPSC can be used to make mini-organs called organoids. These organoids can be used to study disease and treatment in specific tissue types.

CHAPTER 10

Baby is Back!

(A review of cord tissue, placenta, and amniotic fluid/membrane stem cells)

What good mothers and fathers instinctively feel like doing for their babies is usually best after all.
Benjamin Spock

Summary: This chapter reviews the stem cells, which have been discovered in the tissues related to pregnancy, such as the umbilical cord, placenta, and amniotic fluid and membranes, which surround the baby in the uterus. These stem cells are not in routine clinical use, but some clinical trials are underway, which may give us important safety and efficacy information in the future.

STEM CELLS IN TISSUES RELATED TO PREGNANCY

Back in Chapter 3, the development of cord blood stem cell technology and how it has resulted in a great alternative source of 'blood forming' stem cells to treat blood disorders was described. As a result of this excellent work, it soon became apparent that other tissues associated with pregnancy are also potential sources of 'tissue forming' stem cells. These stem cells in tissues related to pregnancy have great potential but also some great challenges.

Umbilical Cord Tissue

The first of these tissues, which were investigated, was the umbilical cord itself, generally known as 'cord tissue'. Cord tissue has been found to contain 'tissue forming' stem cells with the potential to treat a range of diseases already described for 'tissue forming' stem cells. This discovery led private cord blood banks to offer the collection, processing, and storage of cord tissue stem cells to their clients who were already collecting and storing cord blood stem cells. At present, almost all private cord blood clients in the UK and overseas offer to collect and store cord tissue at the time of birth to their clients. The process of collection and storage of cord tissue is easy and it can be carried out by the phlebotomist who collected the cord blood.

Following birth and cord blood collection, a small length of the umbilical cord (usually about 10 cm) is cut and placed into a collection pot provided in the cord blood collection kit. The collection pot contains saline supplemented with antibiotics to minimize bacterial growth in the collected tissue. The cord tissue is then sent to the private cord blood bank laboratory, along with the cord blood, for processing and storage. This, of course, makes more money for private cord blood banks per client and it arguably provides another source of 'tissue forming' stem cells for use in the family. There are, however, some problems with this cord tissue service that rotate around the type, number, and clinical usefulness of cord tissue stem cells.

There is still considerable debate in the scientific community about the nature and number of 'tissue forming' stem cells in the cord tissue. This technical argument is of little interest to the general reader but the outcome of the discussions is that not even the scientists are sure of the type, number, and possible clinical applications of 'tissue forming' stem cells in the cord tissue. This raises questions about the actual potential use of these stem cells and whether or not paying to store them is advisable. The private cord blood banks have, not surprisingly, convincing marketing on this subject but it seems that this marketing bears little resemblance to the current scientific knowledge and evidence. The collection and storage of cord tissue, in parallel with cord blood collection, represents a significant new income source for private cord blood banks. The only people likely to benefit, in the short term at least, are therefore the private cord blood banks.

There is also some variation in the way in which private cord blood banks process and store cord tissue. This could have a big impact on the way in which it might be used in the future. Some private cord blood banks simply cut a small length of the umbilical cord (1-2 cm) into smaller pieces of tissue and freeze the pieces. Other private cord blood banks may process the cord tissue to extract the cord tissue 'tissue forming' stem cells using enzymes and freeze these stem cells. The latter is much cheaper for the cord blood bank than the former and therefore, most cord tissue is stored in small pieces rather than frozen stem cells. This means that if the stem cells are needed, then the tissue must then be thawed and processed to extract the stem cells, which potentially means that the resultant stem cells might be of poor quality or even unsuitable for clinical use. It must also be noted that cord tissue processing to extract stem cells requires the use of enzymes (these are chemicals which speed up biological reactions) to separate the stem cells from the rest of the cord tissue. This, therefore, involves significant manipulation in the eyes of the regulators, which makes the final clinical use of cord tissue stem cells less likely and more expensive to achieve.

Another potential problem with cord tissue 'tissue forming' stem cells is that they are found in relatively low numbers when the cord tissue is broken down using enzymes. This means that to use cord tissue stem cells in any clinical application will almost certainly need an expansion of the cell numbers in the laboratory in order to provide a therapeutic dose. Such expansion is once again another significant manipulation of the cells resulting in increased regulation and increased production costs.

At present, it seems unlikely that cord tissue stem cells will be useful in any routine clinical application in the near future. If they do prove useful, then their preparation for clinical use will be an expensive, time consuming process, and the effort would have to justify the outcome. It would, at present, be much easier to just use fat stem cells. These are readily available and arguably more effective. Despite all of this, private cord blood banks continue to promote the collection and storage of cord tissue and clients continue to pay for the service!

Clinical Trials of Cord Tissue Stem Cells

In terms of the potential clinical applications of cord tissue 'tissue forming' stem cells, there were, at the time of writing, only 4 clinical trials recruiting volunteers using cord tissue stem cells. All four of these clinical trials are looking at diseases which could just as well use 'tissue forming' stem cells from other sources, such as adipose tissue. Therefore, even for clinical trials, these cord tissue stem cells may already be obsolete. On balanced collection and storage of cord tissue, at the time of cord blood collection, is *not worth the investment and private cord blood clients should refuse this service if it is offered.* Public cord blood banks do not collect, process, and store cord tissue for clinical use. If, in the future, the proven clinical utility and safety of cord tissue 'tissue forming' stem cells is demonstrated, then the public cord blood banks could easily begin collection, processing, and storage. I doubt that this will ever happen unless there is a quantum leap in our understanding and use of cord tissue stem cells.

Placenta Stem Cells

The placenta is a complex organ which supplies nutrients and oxygen to a developing baby and removes waste products and carbon dioxide. It functions for the whole of the pregnancy and once delivered after the birth of the baby, it is almost always discarded as medical waste. It has long been part of human cultural and ethnic ceremonies and beliefs, especially in Africa, and indeed some animals will eat the placenta following birth as an important source of nutrients. However, this is not recommended in humans.

Cosmetic companies have, in the past, used the human placenta to develop products that are allegedly anti-aging and generally restorative. There is not much, if any, science behind these claims, but our focus here is stem cell technology and regenerative medicine, not cosmetics.

More recently, the placenta has been shown to contain 'tissue forming' stem cells. It is technically quite difficult to extract these 'tissue forming' stem cells from the placenta because of the size and complexity of the organ. A typical placenta is about the size of a dinner plate and up to two inches (4 cm) thick. The first challenge, therefore, is to develop a suitable container which maintains the placenta at the correct temperature and biological conditions for the journey from the labor ward to the processing laboratory. At present, no such technology exists, but it could easily be developed if interest in placental 'tissue forming' stem cells keeps on increasing.

The second, and perhaps the most difficult, challenge is the safe and effective processing of the placenta to extract stem cells when it arrives in the laboratory. The placenta is a large, fibrous (physically tough) organ requiring a considerable scale-up of processing technology compared to cord tissue. The processing involves dissection of the placenta by a qualified and experienced scientist in clean room (a room with specially filtered air to remove airborne contamination), which is usually followed by some sort of enzyme treatment to break down the placental tissue and thereby release the 'tissue forming' stem cells. This enzyme treatment in the laboratory results in 'significant manipulation' of the stem cells in the eyes of most regulatory authorities, which, in turn, considerably increases the regulatory restrictions and cost placed on placental stem cell use.

Despite all of this, once the placental 'tissue forming' stem cells are obtained, they can easily be frozen for later use. The exact properties of placental 'tissue forming' stem cells have yet to be fully defined. It is likely that they could be useful in regenerative medicine procedures needing stem cells which can make connective tissue, nerves, muscle and potentially many other applications. If we can develop good placenta processing technology, then the number of stem cells obtained from a single placenta will be very high. This will make placental stem cells an attractive source of stem cells for clinical use.

The placenta is also a ready supply of something called the extracellular matrix or ECM. The ECM is a collection of compounds or molecules existing *outside* the cells, which support tissues and organs. It is a sort of biological scaffold holding the cells together. The ECM is extremely important in normal tissue and organ function and is often damaged or destroyed in disease. The fact that the placenta is a good source of ECM makes it even more important in regenerative medicine because stem cells always need a good ECM to do their job properly and the placenta could be an excellent source of this ECM.

The placenta is, therefore, an important potential source of 'tissue forming' stem cells and ECM, but, at present, it is rarely collected apart from some small levels of research. Placental stem cell technology needs research funding and technology development to bring this important source of stem cells and ECM into routinely used regenerative medicine. It should not be discarded as medical waste. There are, at the time of writing, unfortunately no clinical trials using placental stem cells.

Amniotic Membrane and Amniotic Fluid Stem Cells

The amniotic membrane is the membrane which surrounds the baby during development and the amniotic fluid is the fluid surrounding the baby (held in place and produced by the amniotic membrane). The amniotic fluid is usually lost during a normal delivery when the 'waters' break but it is possible to collect it during a Caesarian section. The amniotic membrane is attached to the placenta and can, therefore, easily be collected at most births.

Both amniotic fluid and membrane contain 'tissue forming' stem cells and, therefore, represent a potential source of stem cells for regeneration but they are difficult to collect and do not represent a routine source of 'tissue forming' stem cells.

Clinical Trials of Amniotic Membrane Stem Cells

At the time of writing, there were 3 clinical trials using human amniotic membrane stem cells to treat rejection (GvHD) in 'blood forming' stem cell transplantation. The principle here is that the amniotic membrane stem cells may be able to modulate the immune system of the recipient patient to either reduce or remove the life-threatening symptoms of rejection.

Research and Clinical Trial of Amniotic Membrane Stem Cells

At the time of writing, there was 1 clinical trial assessing the possible use of human amniotic fluid in the treatment of osteoarthritis, tendonitis, and ligament damage. This is based on the ability of 'tissue forming' stem cells to produce the tissues required (cartilage and connective tissue) and also the ability of these stem cells to modulate or reduce inflammation. Inflammation (characterized as being red, swollen, hot, and painful) is the main characteristic and symptom of these conditions and diseases. If the stem cells can reduce inflammation initially, then the likelihood of the stem cells then being able to repair damaged tissue is increased.

There is quite a lot of basic research underway using amniotic membrane in the treatment of burns to the skin and to the eyes. This has been studied using small Phase 1/2 clinical trials, and, whilst much further work is needed, the initial results are very promising and worth pursuing. A similar approach has been selected for using amniotic membrane as a wound dressing in chronic non-healing wounds, such as diabetic ulcers. Once again, the results are very encouraging and further research and development are needed. We are just starting to understand the potential of all of the tissues relating to pregnancy in regenerative medicine and research will bring these to routine clinical use in the years to come.

There are private companies that are working on both amniotic fluid and amniotic membrane technology, but at the time of writing, none of these were at the point of a clinical trial. Their focus, at present, is on initial research and development which is currently ongoing. If such companies can develop products, and take them through a clinical trial, then in the future, we may have safe and effective treatments using amniotic membrane of amniotic fluid stem cells.

KEY POINTS OF CHAPTER 10

- Umbilical cord tissue is a potentially good source of 'tissue forming' stem cells, but much more work is needed to understand the biology of these cells, the numbers of cells needed for treatment and how they may be used in routine clinical practice.
- The stem cells found in the placenta have great future potential but improved collection and processing of the placenta is needed and clinical trials are needed to assess the safety and efficacy of this technology.
- Amniotic membrane and fluid seem to have great potential, especially in the treatment of burns and to assist in wound repair. Much more work is needed to get these concepts into routine clinical use.

CHAPTER 11

Kill or Cure?

(The Controversies Behind Offers of Treatment Made by Stem Cell Companies)

The best cure for insomnia is to get a lot of sleep.
W.C. Fields

Summary: This is perhaps the most important chapter in this book because it offers guidance and advice to patients considering treatment at a private clinic using stem cells and related regenerative medicine technology. This chapter provides information which may help in preventing a lot of pain, suffering, disappointment, and losing a lot of money to rogue stem cell clinics for untested and unproven stem cell-based 'treatments'.

STEM CELL TREATMENTS (*CAVEAT EMPTOR:* BUYER BEWARE*)*

In this book, I have focussed on different stem cell types and on the potential and pros and cons of using these stem cells to treat a very wide range of diseases. There are many pitfalls to avoid stem cell technology, but there are also some promising and exciting ideas, especially at the level of basic laboratory research and future therapies.

There are clearly tried and tested stem cell therapies, such as those involving bone marrow 'blood-forming' stem cells, which have been described in detail. Equally, there are others where the routine clinical applications are either uncertain or even possibly unsafe. The purpose of the previous Chapters was to provide a clear, unbiased opinion on what is currently happening in stem cell technology and regenerative medicine today and empower the reader who may be undergoing or considering undergoing stem cell therapy to remain safe both medically and financially. I hope that I have succeeded to this point and that all readers remain medically and financially safe!

The Regeneration Promise

This chapter is very different and extremely important in the overall discussion of the Regeneration Promise. I now intend to offer specific guidance and advice to anyone considering paying for stem cell treatment for any disease either in your own country, overseas or offshore. There are many private companies worldwide offering stem cell treatments. They are often either located offshore, or in unregulated mainland Countries, and this is usually to avoid the regulatory issues which would otherwise impede their 'treatment' offerings.

These companies typically offer 'treatment' to patients who are most commonly suffering from terminal, degenerative or life-changing disease with no known cure in current medicine. Such potential patients may also be suffering from a debilitating chronic (long-term) disease (for example, diabetic ulcers) with an ineffective treatment in current medicine. Such clinics often list an amazing number of different diseases which they have 'treated' using their technology and support these claims with patient testimonials. This should be seen as the first warning sign. My advice here is that potential patients must be *very* sceptical about such claims and to discuss them with a *trusted* unbiased physician or clinical scientist *before* agreeing to *any* type of treatment.

There are some very important points to consider and to be very cautious about when you are considering a private stem cell clinic:

- If a stem cell company claims that one type of stem cell can treat a wide range of diseases (apart from bone marrow stem cells and blood diseases), then this is at best questionable and at worst irresponsible. They are knowingly trying to mislead. If you see this being promoted by a company, then walk away. There is nothing in the current medical information from clinical trials or basic research, which suggests this wide scope of stem cell technology. Stem cell types, if anything, are disease-specific. Remember: 'The right stem cell for the right job delivered to the right place'.
- If a stem cell company uses patient or celebrity testimonials about their 'treatments', then be extremely cautious about what you believe. Patient or celebrity testimonials may either be fact or fiction (this is impossible to properly assess), and they are most likely to be fiction. Even with an enormous benefit of the doubt, these anecdotal testimonials have little or no relevance or value. Such testimonials (if they are genuine) are simply descriptions of treatment and outcome in an unregulated single treatment event. This does not mean that the treatment discussed is either safe or effective, and it certainly does not recommend that treatment to you. An unethical company (yes, there are unethical stem cell companies!) could even hire actors to make these testimonials, and the viewer has no way of knowing whether it is truth or hoax. Such anecdotal patient testimonials are generally considered to be irrelevant by the medical and scientific community because any beneficial effect maybe just a

coincidence or a spontaneous 'cure' of the disease or the placebo effect or, worse still, a lie. The placebo effect is when a treatment seems to provide benefit even when the active ingredient is removed. It is not well understood and may have a psychological basis. In summary, do not be impressed by patient testimonials under any circumstances. *They cannot be trusted* to be true or relevant to any response you might have to the same 'treatment'.

- Many patients who may be considering stem cell therapy have quite often been through treatments in current medicine, which have either failed or have been ineffective. This means that these patients are very vulnerable. They seek a solution to their problem and many will do anything, including paying large amounts of money, to get access to these 'stem cell or regenerative medicine cures'. This was sadly demonstrated in the recipients of adipose stem cell 'treatment' described in Chapter 8, which resulted in blindness.

If you do decide to talk to a stem cell clinic with a view to some sort of treatment using stem cells and related technology, then there are some key points which you need to be very clear about before proceeding with any agreement; these are:

- You need to trust the clinic you propose to use. This will require you to be critical of *everything* they say and if you do not get satisfactory answers, then do not hesitate to walk away. You should only trust people who are properly qualified and competent to provide healthcare advice. There are many scams and fake qualifications available, which may, at first glance, look impressive but on closer inspection can be either fake or meaningless. You should also assure yourself that not only the 'front-line' people are properly qualified but also those people who support the overall operations in the clinic. If the 'front line' person is a salesman, and the Board consists of businessmen, then be very wary. This means that the clinic is more interested in profit than offering a safe and effective treatment. Please also bear in mind that companies can put almost anything they want to on their own websites, including 'patient' testimonials and 'we are the best'. This information is meaningless and unreliable. If a clinic boasts about being the 'best' then it is a good bet that they are not. Healthcare professionals who are good at their job do not boast that they are the best and that their clinic is better, in fact, they are often the most modest people you can meet. The clinic also needs to have published peer-reviewed publications in medical journals and *unbiased* third party reviews to show that they are professional and trustworthy.
- The subject of money has come up several times in this book. I do not like talking about money and health care, but many people do. Unfortunately, stem cell technology and regenerative medicine is viewed as a simple route to profit by some people. The global regenerative medicine industry is estimated to be

worth $81 billion by 2023! This value of course, includes the good guys and the bad guys. Those companies which operate with an ethical base, and use properly validated, proven and safe regenerative medicine procedures, may find that their treatments are very expensive to provide and profit is therefore small at best. These clinics at least have a good product even if the profit is low.

This of course means that the temptation to take short cuts to a quick profit is very high. Some clinics exist primarily to make money and this potential to make money is vastly increased by frightened, vulnerable patients who, in their desperation, may accept anything a clinic offers. Do not be a victim of such clinics. Some clinics have no real feeling of compassion or duty of care for their patients and if you feel this in discussions with the clinic, then walk away immediately. Be very critical, ask questions and seek second opinions.

- When you receive any proposed costs of treatment, ask for a detailed breakdown of the proposed costs of the treatment and where possible confirm these costs yourself. This might sound difficult but for example if a clinic offers you a specific technique using equipment from a given manufacturer, then contact that manufacturer and find out the list price of the equipment and consumables. If the difference between these costs and the proposed cost of treatment is large then do not be afraid to ask the clinic why this is so? Both good and bad clinics do, of course have overheads and it is not illegal to make a fair profit. It is however unethical (and it should be unlawful) to charge vulnerable patients large amounts for treatments which are either poorly delivered or lack information on safety and effectiveness.
- The clinic itself should be hopefully employing several highly skilled and highly qualified people, so this also has to be put into the cost equation as such expertise and experience does not come cheap. Do not pay any attention to people, such as the Chief Executive Officer (CEO) or any Board member of the clinic for that matter. Such people only have profit in mind. If the clinic has poorly qualified, low skilled people running the clinic or has the CEO as the main point of contact, then not only walk away but also run away!
- It is absolutely essential any clinic you consider for treatment operates to the highest ethical standards. This will help to preserve your safety and well-being. Ethical standards are difficult to quantify, but it can sometimes be judged by the attitude of the staff and the appearance of the clinic itself. It is also perfectly acceptable for you to ask the clinic about which ethical guidelines they work and ask to see a copy of these guidelines. All healthcare professionals work to the highest possible ethical guidelines, but these ethics may not be the focus of the businessmen and investors behind the clinic whose *sole* interest is profit. They do not care at all about you and your illness.

- If you are considering a clinic to provide you with a regenerative medicine or cell therapy treatment, then one of the most important things which you need to see is that the clinic has the appropriate licensing and regulation to carry out the proposed treatment. If the clinic operates in an unregulated or reduced regulatory environment (*e.g.* offshore or in an unregulated mainland Country), then great caution is needed on your part because the clinic can effectively do anything they wish. The level of regulation required by any clinic will vary on the geographical location of the clinic and the nature of the treatments offered by the clinic. For example, any procedure involving cells (taken from one person and given to another person following minimal manipulation) in the UK is licensed and regulated by the HTA (Human Tissue Authority) who issues a 'Human Application' License. The FDA in the USA carries out a similar role. If a regenerative medicine procedure does not involve cells of any type then in the UK the Care Quality Commission (CQC) would oversee and approve the activity in the clinic. Other Countries will have similar organizations. If a clinic uses cells from the patient, carries out minimal manipulation of those cells, and returns them to the same patient on the same day, then this generally does not need specific licensing, but regulatory processes such as CQC approval would be needed.

If the cells which are proposed to be used for treatment are either embryonic stem cells or have undergone significant manipulation in the clinic (*e.g.* iPSC) then this raises the regulatory requirements considerably. Such cells are then considered to be pharmaceutical products and in the UK for example are regulated by the MHRA (Medicines and Healthcare Products Regulatory Agency), which is a higher, more complex level of regulation. All of these regulatory processes are there to protect potential patients, but where regulation is absent, the patient is open to attack.

Other types of accreditation include such things as ISO (International Organisation for Standardisation) which often relates to the operation of the company itself. It does not refer to the quality and safety of cell therapy, meaning that ISO accreditation alone *must not* be accepted as proof of cell therapy regulation by a clinic.

- You must not accept any treatment before you have given informed consent for the treatment. This is a formal process in which those offering the treatment must tell you exactly what the treatment involves, the principles on which the treatment is based, how many people have received the treatment and their outcome or success rates, the risks of the treatment to you and the possible benefits. This process must be carried out by someone qualified to take informed consent (*e.g.* a physician or a clinical scientist), it must be documented and once you are satisfied, both you and the treatment providers must sign the informed consent. You should have the option to have time to consider the informed consent and ask questions before you sign, do not be rushed into signing informed consent. If the people who are offering treatment have inadequate informed consent or no informed consent at all, then walk away.

These basic principles will help you to remain safe when considering regenerative medicine treatments. Do not be afraid to ask questions and to walk away if you have any concerns. There are other points which you also need to be aware of when talking to clinics offering regenerative medicine treatments.

It is also useful to note that in some countries, notably Japan, there is a trend for the regulatory authorities to become more lenient to encourage more investment and activity in stem cell technology. This is contrary to other countries (*e.g.* UK and USA) where regulations are tight, and even increasing, to protect patients. If you live in a Country where stem cell regulations seem to be minimal then please be aware of this and ensure that any treatment offered to you meets international standards of quality and safety. If you are concerned then do not be afraid to ask the clinic involved for more information. Remember, the clinic offering stem cell treatment to you carries a very high duty of care to you.

You may find that some clinics are 'off-shore' (situated on an island) or in countries where regulation is either poor or non-existent. In this situation the clinic can operate with minimum or no regulation and this of course, asks the question as to why this is the case? Some clinics may say that their operations are cheaper and more attractive in a nice location (they may even suggest combining a holiday with your treatment, so-called medical tourism) but of course, the real reason is that they can operate without being overseen by any regulatory authority. Do not consider treatment in any clinic which is 'off-shore' or in a country with poor or no regulation unless their credentials and operations meet international standards. You will be unsafe in such an unregulated clinic; please walk away.

Human Use

In the past, there have been reports of clinics providing treatments using cells or products which are not licensed for human use. This is *extremely dangerous* for the recipient patient. In the UK, for example, all items used for human use (this includes equipment and reagents and in this particular case human cells) must be CE marked in Europe and in the USA FDA approved. This is particularly important if you are considering a treatment where the cells to be used come from a donor. Such donor cells must be collected, processed and stored using technology and reagents, which make them suitable for human use. There are, for example, many excellent companies who supply a range of human stem cells and tissue for *research only*. Such cells and tissue **must not** be used for human treatment and these suppliers make this very clear in their information and product labelling, stating that the product is for research only. Research cells and tissue are cheaper than cells and tissue prepared for clinical use and this encourages some people to think that research grade cells and tissue can be used for clinical use as a cheap alternative. This is wrong and dangerous. If you are considering treatment using donor cells of *any* type, then ask for details of the cells to be used and ensure that the cells are not for research only. Also ensure that the clinic has the necessary regulatory approval for the use of donor cells. Once again, your health and safety is at risk by the use of inappropriate donor cells and if you become concerned then please walk away.

Using Your Own Stem Cells

If your proposed treatment involves using your own cells or tissue (*e.g.* adipose tissue collected from the abdomen or platelet rich plasma PRP from peripheral blood) then this still needs to be carried out safely and meeting regulatory requirements. For example, the processing of your own cells or tissue must take no longer than 4 hours and must not involve any significant manipulation (for example cell culture, use of chemicals such as enzymes or introduction of new genetic material). Such a treatment must always be a 'day-case' *i.e.* everything for a given treatment happens on the same day.

If higher levels of cell or tissue manipulation are needed in your treatment, then your clinic must possess higher levels of regulatory permission. Please be sure to ask these questions about your proposed treatment to ensure your health and safety.

Celebrity Endorsement

Many stem cell clinics spend much more money on marketing than that spent on technology and regulation. This is bad news and a clear sign of a profit-orientated clinic. One area which has seen an increase in the past years is the use of celebrity endorsement. This is a powerful marketing tool as people trust celebrities who they admire *e.g.* a football player or an actor or a pop star. If a celebrity promotes a given stem cell clinic or service, then some people may think that this is a good clinic for that reason. This is, of course, just clever marketing. The celebrity gets paid for their endorsement and the stem cell clinic makes even more profit. If you see a celebrity endorsement, please bear this in mind and remember that such things are simply patient testimonials that are meaningless in terms of the safety and efficacy of any treatment offered.

There is Hope

Finally, a note of re-assurance. There are some excellent clinics in the world offering stem cell and regenerative medicine based treatments which are safe, properly regulated, evidence-based, effective and professional. If you ask the right questions, you will be safe and benefit from the amazing potential of the Regeneration Promise.

KEY POINTS OF CHAPTER 11

- Carry out detailed research and investigation yourself if you are considering stem cell therapy in a private clinic.
- Follow the guidelines provided about the questions to ask a private clinic to ensure your health and safety.
- Do not agree to anything which you either do not fully understand or trust.
- Ensure that regulatory and ethical regulations are observed at all times by the clinic you intend to use.
- Ask questions and if the answers are poor, then walk away.
- Do not be fooled by celebrity endorsements; they do not prove anything.

CHAPTER 12

A Final Thought

(Ideas on cutting edge technology)

Imagination is more important than knowledge. Knowledge is limited. Imagination encircles the world.
Albert Einstein

Summary: This final chapter in this book provides an overview of what is happening at the cutting edge of stem cell and regenerative medicine technology. It describes the research currently underway and how these technologies may have an impact on future clinical practice for all of us. Some of the ideas mentioned here will not be in the public domain, but they are all valid research projects.

SOME THINGS WORK SOME THINGS DO NOT

This is the exciting bit! I can now tell you about some of the amazing ideas for the future of stem cell technology and regenerative medicine. These ideas are all on the very cutting edge of science and medicine and involve concepts which are new, innovative, and sometimes controversial. It is, however, very important to describe these concepts and research because many of them will no doubt find their way, *via* proper evidence-based research and clinical trial, to routine clinical practice in the future. Some of the ideas may fall along the wayside as interesting academic ventures which come to nothing from a practical point of view. This is how all research develops and is not unique to stem cell technology. In science, some things work, some things do not work. If everything works, then that rings many scientific alarm bells. This is the same way that claims about one type of stem cell treating many diseases rings alarm bells. The only exception to this rule is the bone marrow 'blood-forming' stem cell, which can treat 80 different blood disorders. These 80 diseases represent blood disorders and are therefore, one specific group of diseases. It is no surprise that 'blood-forming' stem cells can treat blood disorders.

A mention of any of the technology below *does not* mean that it is either proven or safe, and anyone considering using any of these technologies should initially get advice from a trusted, unbiased physician or clinical scientist before even considering using the technology. This general rule applies to any technology and therapy which has not been thoroughly tested to prove its safety and effectiveness and the aim is to protect people from unsafe and unproven treatments. The technologies are presented in no particular order and an opinion on future importance and possible actions needed for each technology is offered.

Cord Blood Transfusion

In Chapter 3, I described the use of umbilical cord blood as a source 'blood-forming' stem cells to treat leukaemia and blood disorders. Cord blood stem cells are a safe and effective treatment for blood disorders, especially in children. Cord blood can, in fact, also be used in transfusion as a supplement, or alternative to donated adult blood. Donated adult blood is what is commonly known as a blood transfusion around the World.

When cord blood is used for blood transfusion, it can:

• reduce inpatient hospital times
• allow faster recovery and reduce hospital-based deaths for patients suffering from accidents, acute and chronic disease and terminal illness
• Promote a quicker recovery in patients who have had major surgery.

Cord blood transfusion was pioneered by my friend and colleague, Professor Niranjan Bhattacharya, at the Kolkata School of Tropical Medicine.

Umbilical cord blood contains three critical substances which make it much more effective for blood transfusion than donated adult blood, these are:

• Fetal haemoglobin: This is the protein in our red blood cells which carries oxygen. The fetal haemoglobin in cord blood red cells can carry more oxygen than the haemoglobin in donated adult blood red cells. This means that a recipient of a cord blood transfusion, therefore, has higher oxygenation rates than the recipient of donated adult blood. This could be critical in severe illness, trauma, or during and after surgery where patients often suffer from low oxygen levels.
• Cytokines (proteins) which are not present in donated adult blood. These can reduce the damage caused by trauma and disease and promote faster recovery rates for these patients
• Stem cells (both blood-forming and tissue-forming) may help to repair damaged tissue in both accidents and disease

Cord blood for transfusion would be collected as described in Chapter 3 and grouped (using the standard ABO blood group system) and screened for infectious disease in the same way as donated adult blood. Most Countries have the infrastructure needed for this process.

Professor Bhattacharya has carried out hundreds, possibly now thousands, of cord blood transfusions in India and found no adverse effects at all in these recipients. We must not ignore this priceless resource and related technology. At present, 99% of potential cord blood donations are discarded as medical waste and we should, in my opinion, start to think about cord blood not only for transplantation but also for transfusion.

Most major hospitals have a labour ward, and they have lots of patients who need blood transfusion. Such hospitals also have A&E and surgical or oncology departments with constant demands for blood for transfusion. Cord blood could be collected in the labour ward and then easily used as a reliable and effective transfusion product for their patients in the same hospital. A large labour ward could potentially provide the transfusion needs for the whole hospital and even more.

NHSBT (the blood and transplant section of the NHS) and equivalent organizations globally often warn of donated adult blood shortages; these are mainly seasonal shortages. This approach to the collection of cord blood for transfusion could not only remove these shortages but also save the health care providers a considerable amount of time and money and reduce a significant amount of suffering in our patient population.

Using cord blood for transfusion is a fantastic idea, but as with all of these 'cutting edge' technologies, we must proceed with caution to ensure that no one suffers along the way. The next step is to bring cord blood transfusion into use in a small number of patients (a phase I clinical to trial) to ensure safety, and if this turns out to be so (which is what Professor Bhattacharya has already shown), then the technology could then be brought into general use in Phase II multi-center clinical trial. If we can bring umbilical cord blood transfusion into routine clinical practice it could be a lifesaver and it could also revolutionize the way in which we understand and use blood transfusion.

Cord blood transfusion could also be extremely useful in Countries where the infrastructure for adult blood donation is either poor on non-existent. In this context, I am currently working with colleagues in Nigeria to bring cord blood transfusion to Nigerian hospitals.

Platelet Rich Plasma (PRP)

We all have platelets (small particles which promote blood clotting when needed) in our blood. Platelet rich plasma (PRP) is a technology which concentrates these platelets, which can then be used clinically to treat painful joints and muscles, to promote wound healing, and in many other applications, which are in clinical trial.

The process of collecting and preparing PRP is relatively simple. Around 20-30mL of venous blood is collected and then centrifuged in a special PRP tube which separates the cells from the PRP. The PRP is usually produced from the patient who is seeking treatment *i.e.* it is an autologous procedure using the patients' own blood with minimum manipulation. PRP therefore, it attracts very little attention in terms of regulatory authorities.

The PRP can then be taken and used in whatever way is needed. Since this is a very simple process, almost any clinic or laboratory could produce PRP and offer it as a treatment route. The 'rogue' clinics have started to offer this treatment as a therapy for almost everything!

PRP is interesting and certainly worth more research and clinical trials. It is not a routine treatment, and it should not be offered as such. If you are interested in PRP therapy, then the best advice is to join one of the 89 and counting clinical trials around the World. Do not pay for PRP treatment in private clinics unless they have excellent safety and effectiveness data.

Very Small Embryonic Like Stem Cells and Laser Technology

One of the most exciting areas of clinical research in regenerative medicine is an area called photoacoustic therapy. This is the impact of light and sound on biological systems and especially stem cells. One of the leading pioneers of this technology is Dr. Todd Ovokaitys (known to his friends and colleagues as Dr. Todd) based at a company called Qigenix in California. Dr. Todd and his colleagues have developed a medical laser, which produces specially modulated laser light, which appears to 'stimulate' or 'activate' stem cells to carry out repair more quickly and more efficiently than without exposure to the laser. The laser also seems capable of directing stem cells to where they are needed in the body to carry out repair and regeneration. This is achieved by applying the laser (which is a totally harmless low energy red laser especially modulated for this application) to the patient in the area where the repair is needed *e.g.* to the area of the heart in heart disease and so on.

This research and development using the laser have focused on a group of stem cells known as Very Small Embryonic Like (VSEL) stem cells, which have not been mentioned so far in this book. There was initially some debate about whether or not these VSEL stem cells actually existed but they have now clearly been identified in peripheral blood in the veins of us all and in many other organs and tissues in the body. They are called VSEL stem cells because they are very small (diameter of 1-4 millionth of a metre) and have similar surface markers as embryonic stem cells discussed in Chapter 6.

It is proposed that VSEL stem cells are 'tissue forming' stem cells in the same way as embryonic stem cells and therefore theoretically capable of making any of the different tissues and cells in the body. These VSEL stem cells are found in everyone in our circulating blood, but in normal circumstances they seem to be biologically inactive. It is thought that VSEL stem cells may be a remnant of our biological development, which were active in the developing fetus but become no longer active shortly after birth and for the rest of a persons' life. There is also a thought that as VSEL stem cells are found in the bone marrow, they may be responsible for creating the 'blood-forming' stem cells found in the bone marrow. This has yet to be confirmed, but it seems likely that this may be happening. A lot more research is needed on this subject.

The best and easiest way to isolate these VSEL stem cells is to collect some peripheral blood from a vein and process it in a centrifuge to produce a fraction of the blood known as platelet-rich plasma (PRP) as described above. This PRP fraction contains high numbers of platelets (components of the blood involved in blood clotting) and also high numbers of VSEL stem cells. The next step in the process is to shine the modulated red light medical laser at the PRP for about 3 minutes in total to 'activate' the VSEL stem cells, which can then be returned to the patient to either a specific site, *e.g.* the knee joint or a specific organ or back into a vein. The laser can then also be applied to the area where treatment is needed to attract the stem cells to where they are needed and instruct them to remain in that area.

The fact that VSEL stem cells are very small means that if they are returned into the patient into a vein then they are small enough to get to any site in the body, including the brain. This is not the case with other stem cell types such as standard 'tissue forming' stem cells, which, if injected into a vein will almost all be caught up in the tiny blood vessels in the lung.

My own research on VSEL stem cells, in collaboration with Dr Todd, has shown that when the modulated laser is used on PRP (VSEL stem cells) it causes the VSEL stem cells to increase in number very rapidly and this could be part of the 'activation' process. The full mechanism of the 'activation' process is still in the research laboratory so watch this space!

Dr Todd has a lot of data from a Phase I clinical trial and patient case studies on the clinical use of 'activated' VSEL stem cells. This includes the use of activated VSEL stem cells in the treatment of neurological disease (*e.g.* Parkinson's disease and multiple sclerosis) in nerve damage (*e.g.* spinal damage following an accident or injury) and in a clinical trial using 'activated' VSEL stem cells to treat life-threatening heart failure. Patients in these and many other groups seem to benefit from 'activated' VSEL stem cell therapy. In the heart failure clinical trial, all patients seemed to benefit from the treatment which helped them all to resume a normal life and the benefits seem to be stable over time.

Laser activated VSEL stem cell therapy is not a 'cure'. No such claims have ever been made. Nevertheless, laser activated VSEL stem cell therapy does seem to be a benefit to many patients in terms of increasing their quality of life. It appears that the most benefit is seen when the treatment is used in the early stages of disease or trauma, but once again more work is needed to confirm this observation. It may well be true based on the fact that scar and fibrous tissue is common in persistent disease but is not so common at the start of the disease. The scar and fibrous tissue may be reducing the effectiveness of any stem cell therapy. The benefit of laser activated VSEL stem cells is also enhanced when the patient is treated in a holistic way *i.e.* combining all the things the patient needs rather than just an injection of stem cells. Much more basic scientific research and further detailed clinical trials are needed on this technology but it is an area of great excitement in regenerative medicine which certainly deserves a mention in this book. It has the potential to make an enormous contribution to the Regeneration Promise in the future, but only time will tell.

Cell Reprogramming

In Chapter 9, I described the development of induced pluripotent stem cells (iPSC) and their possible uses in regenerative medicine. Researchers have in fact, already moved on from this initial idea to the concept of 'reprogramming' normal cells not only to iPSC but also directly to the cell of interest. In normal iPSC technology, once the iPSC is created, it is then treated in various ways to obtain the cell actually needed for use *e.g.* some heart cells. A company in Cambridge, UK called Mogrify is developing technology which will enable us to 'reprogramme' a normal cell (*e.g.* a skin cell) directly to the cell required to use in regenerative medicine procedures. They therefore, 'transmogrify' the cells and hence the company name. The benefit of this is that instead of the process being multi-step with the opportunity for problems along the way, the process will be a single step to obtain the cells required for clinical use. This approach could make iPSC obsolete, but it could also provide us with easily produced cells for regenerative medicine procedures. There is still a lot to do to bring this to routine clinical practice through clinical trials but it is a great idea which may have a big part to play in the Regeneration Promise in the future.

Exosomes

An area of cell biology which is attracting a lot of research at present is a subject called exosomes. Exosomes are tiny packets of information released by cells, approximately 30 to 100 billionth of a meter in diameter, which is thought to be involved in cell to cell communication and in cell to cell regulation. There is also some thought that exosomes may be a useful way to deliver drugs in the future, but at present, this is just a concept and not a reality. The very small size of exosomes, most of which are in the same size range as viruses, make them relatively difficult to isolate and manipulate, but many researchers are making good progress with isolation technology, which is helping in the proper understanding. Nevertheless, at present, we are in the very early stages of understanding exosomes in terms of what they do in normal life and how they may be manipulated in the future in therapeutic use. Despite this very early stage of understanding exosome technology, there are some commercial companies who try to sell exosome technology to unsuspecting patients suffering from a very wide range of diseases. These companies are irresponsible since we do not, at present, even understand the basic biology of exosomes and exosomes; therefore cannot and must not be offered for clinical use. The safety and effectiveness of exosomes are currently unknown. At the time of writing, there were 26 clinical trials recruiting volunteers for a wide range of clinical trials assessing the possible use of exosomes in malignancies to various types of gum inflammation. Patients can of course, offer to take part in such clinical trials but bear in mind that such volunteers should never be asked to pay to take part in the clinical trial. Any private company offering exosome therapy to patients for a fee is offering technology in which safety and efficacy have not been proven. Take care!

Quantum Medicine

The subject of quantum medicine is relatively new and very difficult to understand, even for those with a good grasp of science and medicine. It actually lends itself to be understood best by physicists.

Quantum medicine involves the description of normal physiological activity, disease states and even novel therapeutic strategies based on the activity of sub-atomic particles, which are the smallest things we know to exist. These particles are described by the branch of physics called quantum mechanics. If this level of understanding and application can be reached, and it might take decades to do so, then it will revolutionize the way in which we think about disease and therapy. There have already been some advances where teams have described the sense of smell in quantum terms and also, the amazing ability of some birds to return to the correct place at the correct time may have a quantum basis. Even photosynthesis (energy formation in plants derived from light) is thought to have a basis in quantum biology. Eventually, we may be able to describe everything in medicine in quantum terms, which will enable better therapy and outcomes for the whole of the human race. The important thing to stress is that a full understanding of quantum medicine is an extremely demanding, time-consuming and no doubt expensive process which will not appear in routine clinical practice for decades and perhaps not at all if our understanding and technical abilities do not meet the challenge. If anyone invokes ideas about quantum medicine, and claims to have it available for use now, then they are opportunistic cheats who are just trying to cash in on vulnerable patients. Quantum medicine has enormous potential, but it will take considerable time and more research and understanding before it can be applied to everyday thinking and therapy.

Nanotechnology

Nanotechnology is the production of extremely small products which can have innovative uses across the whole of science and medicine. Perhaps the most famous of these is a substance called graphene, which is a single layer of carbon atoms arranged in a hexagonal lattice. Graphene, and other nanomaterials, can be used as a support system for stem cells because it is known that stem cells function better if they are supported and can form what is known as a microenvironment. The microenvironment is extremely important to the long-term survival and action of stem cells.

The use of nanomaterials in combination with stem cells has shown great promise in the fields of neurology (treating diseases associated with the central nervous system) and treatments for the repair of bone in both disease and trauma.

There is clearly an enormous clinical potential in this area of biotechnology, which brings together clinical scientists, physicists, biotechnologists, physicians, biotechnology companies and all other related professions to create successful research and development of this technology. Much of the data at present are experimental but encouraging. In the future, we need to develop and carry out clinical trials to demonstrate the safety and efficacy of nanotechnology in regenerative medicine. Once these trials are safely and effectively completed, this will lead to the introduction of nanotechnology into routine clinical practice, which will also enable the long-term epidemiology of the technology to be assessed.

An important factor in the use of nanomaterials in regenerative medicine will be the source and type of stem cells used in conjunction with nanomaterials. This could be from the patient himself such as Very Small Embryonic Like stem cells (VSEL), which are easily collected from the peripheral blood. Laser activation of VSEL, to make VSEL into active cells could be an excellent partner for nanomaterials. Another tissue which could be used from the patient is fat tissue stem cells which are easily collected from the patient and, with non-enzymatic processing technology, can be collected and processed as and when required by the patient. It is also possible to use donated 'tissue forming' stem cells with nanomaterials and such cells have the added advantage that they can be transplanted without concern for rejection by the recipient patient. Such 'tissue forming' stem cells could be collected from donors, processed, frozen and released for patient use when required. A more complex approach could include the use of induced pluripotent stem cells (iPSC).

Research is needed to evaluate whether patient derived or donor stem cells are the best choice of stem cells to combine with nanomaterials. It is likely that each different disease or trauma calls for a different nanomaterial/stem cell combination which is why it is important to keep an open mind on which is the best way to proceed. Whatever happens, any future nanomaterial/stem cell therapy must be evidence-based and supported by clear beneficial data from clinical trials.

This final step, bringing the nanotechnology into routine clinical practice, will need careful regulatory input to ensure that the correct policies and procedures are utilized to protect patients and that the new nanotechnology medical devices are manufactured and tested to the highest possible standards. The production of stem cells for nanomaterial use will need national and international regulation to ensure safety and best practice, as will the nanomaterials which will be categorised as medical devices. This combination of innovation, collaboration, basic research and clinical trial using nanotechnology will open up a new era in the treatment of many diseases and injuries.

3D Printing

3D printing is technology which allows the production of a three-dimensional object using data in a computer to drive the process. These data could, for example, be a laser scan of a heart valve which then drives the printing of a heart valve. This has many applications in general manufacturing and the technology is now being used to create structures on which stem cells can grow. Examples of using this approach to enable stem cells to be used in novel clinical applications include the creation of 'patches' to repair heart tissue and structures such as heart valves and major blood vessels, which can be covered in tissue produced from stem cells. A similar approach has been used to develop patches of skeletal muscle tissue which also have the potential to repair damaged muscle resulting from trauma or disease and also to create patches of liver and skin tissue with a similar intention to use in liver and skin disease and injury.

This technology has great potential, especially in organ regeneration, but we are still learning and much more research needs to be carried out in order to fully understand the possibilities. The challenges which need to be solved include how the patches of tissue would obtain a sufficient blood flow to ensure that the tissue remains healthy as it grows and develops in the body, to optimise the material from which the 3D object is printed and most importantly, to develop highly regulated and controlled procedures in 3D printing for clinical use.

Skeletal Muscle Stem Cells

There has been a lot of research on stem cells found in muscle, especially skeletal muscle, which are the muscles which allow normal movement. This is providing excitement and optimism about potential therapies using such cells. Muscle repair is needed in a variety of diseases and situations such as acute disease, which results in muscle wasting, a genetic disease such as muscular dystrophy, which leads to long-term muscle deterioration and death and trauma to muscle. At present, the rebuilding of muscle in these situations is based on on physiotherapy and exercise, but the inclusion of a muscle-based stem cell in the treatment of such patients may speed recovery. There is still much to do in this field, but the coming years will no doubt see clinical trials and eventually routine procedures which use muscle stem cells.

Liver Stem Cells

The liver is an organ which is known to be able to regenerate from damage in certain circumstances. This may be following the donation of a part of the liver for transplant or recovery of the liver following trauma or poisoning from alcohol or drugs. In the case of alcohol or drug damage it is essential that alcohol and drug use stop before there is any possibility of regeneration and in many cases, such livers are damaged beyond repair. This ability to repair indicates that there must be stem cells in the liver, which are active throughout our lives, which can repair the liver in some circumstances. It therefore follows that it may be possible to extract stem cells from the liver and use them as a source of stem cells for regenerative protocols for the liver. Once again, this is very much in the research phase at present and will no doubt go to clinical trial and routine therapy in the future.

Recent Progress in Stem Cell Therapy of Heart Disease

The point that 'the right stem cell for the right job' is needed has been made clearer recently by some success using umbilical cord-derived 'tissue-forming' stem cells to treat heart failure . In this work, researchers gave 'tissue forming'

stem cells into the vein of heart failure patients and the patients showed some benefits following treatment in terms of improved heart function.

This approach of giving 'tissue forming' stem cells into a vein and expecting them to get into the heart (or any specific organ for that matter) is, in my opinion (and that of many others) flawed. This is because when 'tissue-forming' stem cells are injected into a vein most, if not all of them, will be trapped in tiny blood vessels in the lungs. This is because 'tissue forming' stem cells are simply too large to pass through the lungs without getting trapped. The benefits are observed in the introduction of 'tissue-forming' stem cells described above may possibly be due to chemicals secreted by the 'tissue-forming' cells acting on the heart or possibly from exosomes (tiny packets of cellular material) produced by the 'tissue forming' stem cells which could easily find their way to the heart.

A better approach in getting 'tissue forming' stem cells to the heart is to use a cardiac catheter to place the stem cells exactly where they are needed in the heart. This work is in the research and development phase just now, but the approach is likely to improve patient outcomes and it will also enable the delivery of stem cells directly to other organs in the future. In the light of this type of work, the 'right stem cell for the right job' should perhaps be revised to the 'right stem cell for the right job delivered in the right way'.

Anti-Ageing

Over the years, there have been many claims that a certain drug or cosmetic can achieve anti-aging. Most of these claims are either false or at best misleading and often, the evidence (most commonly a 'before' and 'after' photograph) is at best unconvincing. There is, however, a clear biological reason for ageing and it is related to the ageing of our stem cells. It is good to recall that stem cells are the basis of the maintenance of organs such as bone marrow, skin and the gastrointestinal tract. Daily repair of these tissues enables normal healthy life. As stem cells age, they become less efficient and therefore, the daily repair they provide decreases in quality and effectiveness. This can be very clearly seen in the ageing of skin, which is a direct result of the ageing of skin stem cells.

Every cell (apart from red cells in the blood which have no nucleus) in our body contains DNA and each piece of DNA has a section on the end of each strand known scientifically as a telomere. Every time a cell divides during our lifetime, the length of the telomere decreases and when the telomere is totally gone then, the cell dies. This reduction in telomere length in stem cells as they divide is the basis of ageing of our major organs and tissues. It therefore follows that if we can increase or stabilize the telomere length, then ageing would either be halted or stopped. There have been many attempts to intervene in telomere shortening, but at the moment there are no convincing and safe procedures which can achieve this goal.

On the premise that ageing of the body is related to ageing of the stem cells in that body, then some people have proposed that if we introduce 'younger' stem cells with long telomeres then this may halt or delay ageing. In theory, this is a good idea, stem cells could, for example, be used from umbilical cord blood or umbilical cord tissue as a source of young, long telomere stem cells. If such stem cells could be directed to repair such tissue as skin, then this could, in theory, produce an anti-ageing effect in the recipient patient. This is an interesting concept which will need much further research but will no doubt come into use in the future. We must however be clear that ageing is a natural process essential to the long term survival of the human race. If science stops ageing then the consequences for humans and planet Earth could be catastrophic.

The Regeneration Promise is sometimes amazing, sometimes disappointing, sometimes frustrating, sometimes astonishing, but it is always inspirational. The things described in the chapter are 'cutting-edge' science, which will hopefully come to reality one day in terms of a safe and reliable treatment for some of the most destructive illnesses and shocking trauma imaginable.

A Final Thought

I hope that you have enjoyed this book. It has been my mission for many years to bring the world of stem cell technology to everyone who either needs to know or just has a general interest. I want to dispel the fears, clear up the hype, and to show that underneath all of this that there is a technology which will help millions of people for generations to come. Regenerative Medicine will eventually be a routine in hospitals around the World and we will wonder how we ever managed without it. I hope that you found the book informative, educational and even funny in places. I tried my best, I am after all a scientist not a comedian!

Stem cell technology has been my life's work. From my totally absorbing Ph.D. with Bob Edwards in Cambridge working on basic ideas in 'blood forming' stem cells, to my most recent work on the use of laser technology and quantum physics to attempt to explain what might be happening when laser light hits a stem cell. This technology may be able to activate and use Very Small Embryonic Like

(VSEL) stem cells for therapy. These are cells in everyone and which may have otherwise been dormant since birth. This really 'shines a light' on stem cell technology!

Over that time, I have carried out clinical work in stem cell technology and assisted reproduction, university teaching, basic research, clinical research and worked in the NHS and the private sector. I have worked in Europe, N. America and Nigeria. I have met (and continue to meet) some fantastic people who have

the same vision as me and the whole trip has been, and is, amazing. I could not have wished for a better career or a better life, and I thank everyone involved.

In some ways, this book is the pinnacle of my work and career and in others, it is just an important stepping-stone to other things. If it helps and advises current and future people who are considering some sort of stem cell technology treatment, either for themselves or for a family member, then my job is done. If not, I have failed, but that's another story…

In its final passage, a good book does not require understanding; but rather the understanding of the book's main idea.

Alan Maiccon

KEY POINTS OF CHAPTER 12

- Stem cell technology is developing very rapidly, but it is still in its infancy
- Some novel ideas will work, others will not
- Keep an open mind but do not be drawn into areas where the evidence is weak or non-existent; the whole of science must be evidence-based
- If you are a young scientist tempted to get into Regenerative Medicine, then do not hesitate!

SUGGESTED FURTHER READING

- A Matter of Life (1980) by Robert G. Edwards & Patrick C. Steptoe. Hutchinson Books.
- Life before Birth (1989) by Robert G. Edwards. Hutchinson Books.

USEFUL LINKS

- https://www.mssociety.org.uk/about-ms/treatments-and-therapies/dise-se-modifying-therapies/hsct/hsct--what-to-expect
- http://www.aabb.org/aabbcct/therapyfacts/Pages/default.aspx
- https://www.anthonynolan.org/patients-and-families

- https://www.bioeden.com/uk/
- https://www.cqc.org.uk/
- https://clinicaltrials.gov/
- https://www.closerlookatstemcells.org/
- https://www.ebmt.org/jacie-accreditation
- http://www.factwebsite.org/
- https://www.fda.gov/home
- https://media.nature.com/original/magazine-assets/d41586-019-02-82-0/d41586-019-02882-0.pdf
- https://www.mssociety.org.uk/about-ms/treatments-and-therapies/dise-se-modifying-therapies/hsct/hsct--what-to-expect
- https://stemcellsportal.com/press-releases/induced-pluripotent-stem-cells-show-success-treating-hemophilia-mice
- https://www.iso.org/standards.html
- https://www.livescience.com/58287-unproven-stem-cell-therapy-blindness.html
- https://www.gov.uk/government/organisations/medicines-and-healthca-e-products-regulatory-agency
- https://mogrify.co.uk/technology/#our-science
- https://nyscf.org/
- https://parentsguidecordblood.org/en
- http://qigenix.com/
- http://www.stmkolkata.org/rmts/head-of-department%20.html

GLOSSARY

Autologous: This is a treatment where cells or tissue are taken from a patient processed and returned to the same patient

Allogeneic: This is a treatment where cells or tissue are obtained from a donor and given to an unrelated recipient. The donor cells are often frozen before use.

'Blood Forming' Stem Cells: These are stem cells found in the bone marrow and cord blood. Bone marrow blood forming stem cells can be mobilised into the circulation as peripheral blood stem cells using medication for easier collection. The scientific name for these stem cells is haemopoietic stem cells.

Cell Programming: This is technology which can enable the transformation of normal body cells (*e.g.* skin cells) directly into the cells needed for treatment (*e.g.* heart cells) by introducing the precise growth factors and genes needed for the direct cell transformation. This is a refined form of induced pluripotent stem cells which instead of going to the stem cell state the method allows direct transformation to the target cell state.

Cord Blood Stem Cells: These are blood forming stem cells which can be isolated from the blood remaining in the umbilical cord and placenta at the birth of a baby.

Cord Blood Transfusion: This is the use of whole cord blood collected at birth as an alternative or supplement to donated adult blood. Cord blood transfusion may have benefits over adult blood transfusion and could be used in parallel to adult blood transfusion.

Cord Blood Transplantation: This is the process by which cord blood stem cells are used to treat blood disorders.

Cord Blood Unit: A cord blood unit is the frozen stem cells collected from a cord blood collection which are stored frozen in liquid nitrogen in a bag about the size of a credit card. The cord blood unit is what is sent frozen to the hospital for transplantation.

Dental Pulp Stem Cells: These are the 'tissue forming' stem cells found inside baby and adult teeth. The stem cells can be collected and frozen for later use.

Fat (adipose) Stem Cells: These are stem cells found in fat (*e.g.* fat from the abdomen). They are known scientifically as adipose stem cells and they are 'tissue forming' or mesenchymal stem cells.

Haemopoietic Stem Cells: This is the scientific name for 'blood forming' stem cells found in bone marrow and cord blood.

Human Tissue Authority (HTA): This is the UK regulatory authority which regulates the use of human cells in procedures such as bone marrow transplantation and cell therapy

Induced Pluripotent Stem Cells: These are 'man made' stem cells created by inserting new genetic material (genes) into normal body cells such as skin cells.

Mesenchymal Stem Cells: This is the scientific name for 'tissue forming' stem cells.

Organoids: These are tight ball like collections of cells derived from induced pluripotent stem cells, which can be formed into most tissues of the body. They provide a potential system to study development, organ physiology and possible drug testing.

Public Cord Blood bank: This is a cord blood collection processing and storage facility usually run by a healthcare provider *e.g.* in the UK the NHS Blood and Tissue Service (NHSBT). These organisations collect cord blood, process it and store it and make it available to anyone in need. The donor does not pay for this process and the public cord blood bank will charge the recipient hospital when providing a cord blood unit for transplant.

Pluripotent Stem Cells: These are stem cells found in developing human and animal embryos, which have the potential to form all tissues in the body.

Private Cord Blood Bank: This is a company which provides cord blood collection processing and storage for family use only and an initial fee and an annual storage fee is paid for this service.

Teeth Stem Cells: These are stem cells found inside adult and infant teeth which can be collected and stored frozen. Teeth cells (known scientifically as dental pulp stem cells) are 'tissue forming' or mesenchymal stem cells.

Telomere: A portion of DNA on the end of each chromosome which reduces as the cell divides and undergoes ageing.

'Tissue Forming' Stem Cells: These are stem cells found in the umbilical cord tissue placenta, fat and teeth. They are also present, but in lower numbers, in bone marrow. They are known scientifically as mesenchymal stem cells.

SUBJECT INDEX

www.ingramcontent.com/pod-product-compliance
Lightning Source LLC
Chambersburg PA
CBHW060801270326
41926CB00002B/52